AF365184

Physical Pharmaceutics-II

Physical Pharmaceutics-II

Suryadevara Vidyadhara

Professor and Principal,

Janga Ramesh Babu

M.Pharm., Ph.D

Professor,

Department of Pharmaceutics

Chebrolu Hanumaiah Institute of Pharmaceutical Sciences,

(Formerly N.E.S. Institute of Pharmaceutical Sciences),

Chandramoulipuram, Chowdavaram, Guntur-522 019.

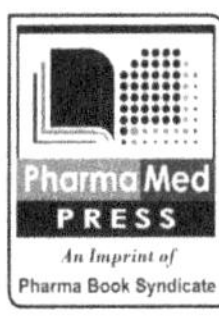

PharmaMed Press

An imprint of Pharma Book Syndicate

A Unit of BSP Books Pvt. Ltd.

4-4-309/316, Giriraj Lane,

Sultan Bazar, Hyderabad - 500 095.

Physical Pharmaceutics-II *by Suryadevara Vidyadhara and Janga Ramesh Babu*

© 2016, *by Publisher*

Published by

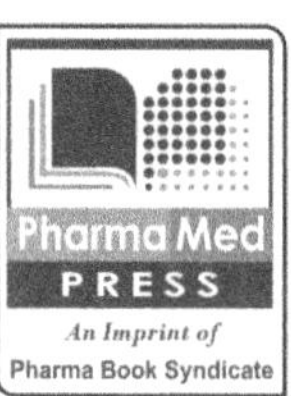

PharmaMed Press

An imprint of Pharma Book Syndicate

A unit of BSP Books Pvt. Ltd.

4-4-309/316, Giriraj Lane, Sultan Bazar, Hyderabad - 500 095.

Phone: 040-23445605, 23445688; Fax: 91+40-23445611

e-mail: info@pharmamedpress.com

ISBN: 978-93-5230-112-6 (HB)

PREFACE

The authors are pleased to bring out the first edition of Physical Pharmaceutics-II. This book is written specially to provide the coverage of syllabus for students of both undergraduate and post graduate level in the subject of physical Pharmacy. The subject of physical pharmacy has been associated with basics of pharmaceutics and gives idea about theoretical principles which can be applied in the formulation development of any dosage form.

This book contains eight chapters which covers the syllabus of the most of the Indian universities. The salient feature of this book is the presentation of fundamental concepts in a very simplified and self explanatory form. It is expected that present textbook of physical Pharmaceutics-II would facilitate in laying a sound foundation in students for pharmaceutics.

The authors are grateful to the management of Nagarjuna Education Society (NES) and Chebrolu Hanumaiah Institute of Pharmaceutical Sciences (CHIPS) Guntur, for constant encouragement provided during completion of this book.

The authors would like to thank to all the faculty members and students of CHIPS, friends and family members who have been the source of inspiration in the preparation of this book.

The authors express sincere thanks to PharmaMed Press for kind co-operation and immense interest taken in bringing out this book.

The authors have made every attempt, strived hard to present a good book. The authors would appreciate any suggestions from students, fellow teachers and research scholars for future improvement of this book.

Dr. S. Vidyadhara

Dr. J. Ramesh Babu

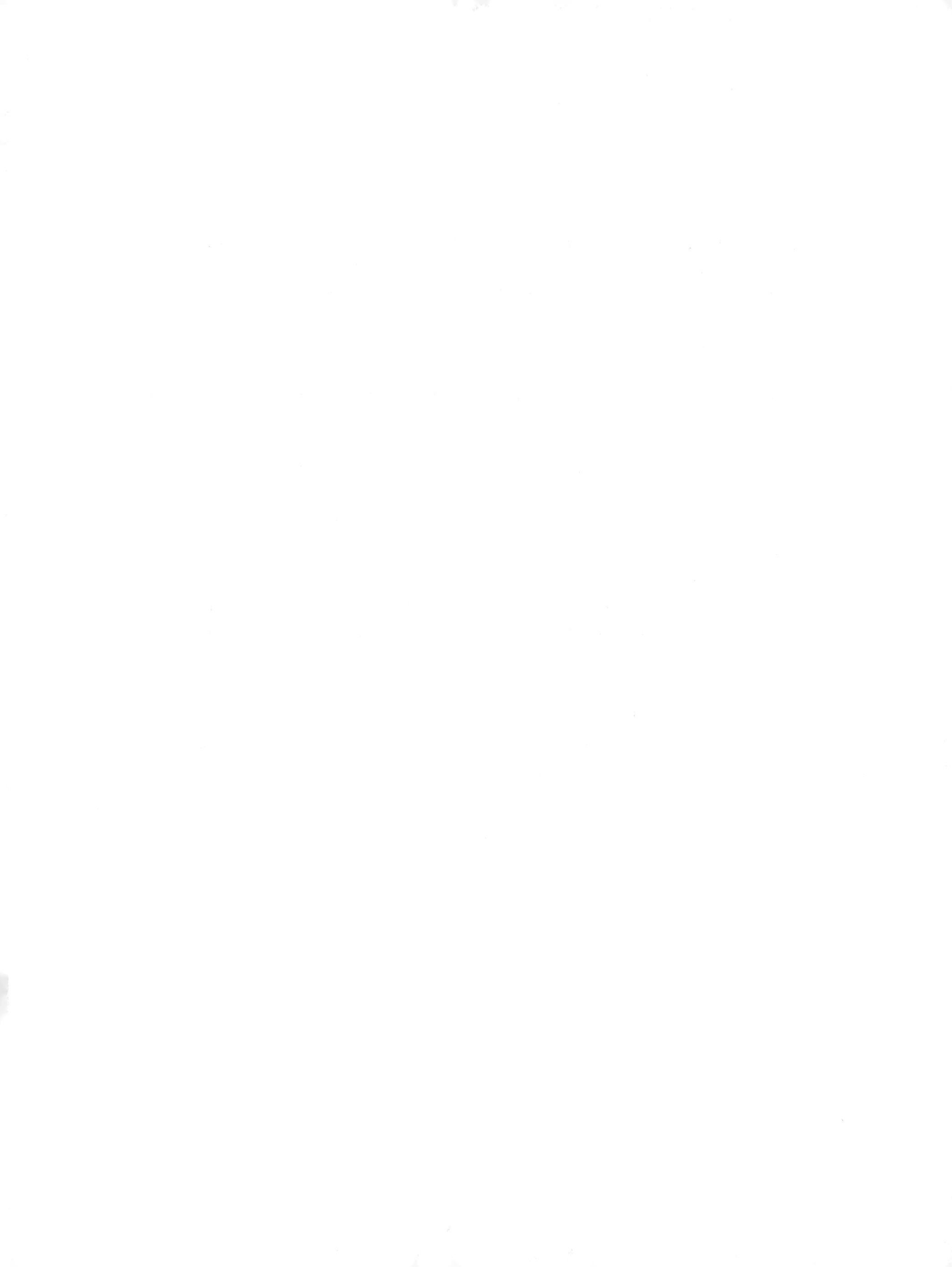

CONTENTS

Preface ....(v)

Chapter 1A

Solubility

1A.1 Introduction 1

  1A.1.1 Definition of Terms.. 1

  1A.1.2 Methods of Expressing Solubility.................................... 1

1A.2 Solute-Solvent Interactions 2

  1A.2.1 Polar Solvents 2

  1A.2.2 Non Polar Solvents 3

  1A.2.3 Semi Polar Solvents 3

1A.3 Ideal and Real Solutions.. 3

1A.4 Solubility of Gases In Liquids... 6

  1A.4.1 Factors Affecting Solubility of Gases in Liquids............. 6

1A.5 Solubility of Liquids in Liquids 7

  1A.5.1 Factors Affecting Solubility of Liquids in Liquids 8

1A.6 Solubility of Solids in Liquids.. 11

  1A.6.1 Solubility of Solids in Liquids Determination 11

  1A.6.2 Factors Affecting Solubility of Solids in Liquids 13

1A.7 Solubility of Strong Electrolytes 16

1A.8 Solubility of Slightly Soluble Electrolytes 17

1A.9 Solubility of Weak Electrolytes.. 18

Chapter 1B

Distribution Phenomena

1B.1 Introduction 20

1B.2 Partition Coefficient 20

  1B.2.1 Effect of Partition of Ionic Dissociation and
      Molecular Association 21

  1B.2.2 Extraction.. 24

1B.3 Solubility and Partition Coefficients 25

  1B.3.1 Preservative Action of Weak Acids in Oil-Water Systems...... 25

1B.4 Drug Action and Partition Coefficients 27

Chapter 1C

Fick's Laws of Diffusion

1C.1   Introduction 28

    1C.1.1   Drug Absorption and Elimination 28

    1C.1.2   Drug Release 29

    1C.1.3   Osmosis 29

    1C.1.4   Ultra Filtration and Dialysis 29

1C.2   Steady-State Diffusion 29

    1C.2.1   Thermodynamic Basis 29

1C.3   Fick's Laws of Diffusion 31

    1C.3.1   Fick's First Law 31

    1C.3.2   Fick's Second Law 31

Chapter 2

Complexation

2.1   Definition 34

    2.1.1   Classification of Complexes 34

2.2   Metal Ion Complexes 35

    2.2.1   Inorganic Complexes 35

    2.2.2   Chelates 36

    2.2.3   Olefin and Aromatic Type 37

2.3   Organic Molecular Complexes 37

    2.3.1   Donor-Acceptor Type 37

    2.3.2   Charge Transfer Complexes 38

    2.3.3   Drug and Caffeine Complexes 38

    2.3.4   Polymer Complexes 39

    2.3.5   Picric Acid Complexes 39

    2.3.6   Quinhydrone Complexes 40

2.4   Inclusion Complexes 40

    2.4.1   Channel Lattice Type 40

    2.4.2   Layer Types 41

    2.4.3   Clathrates 41

    2.4.4   Monomolecular Inclusion Complexes 42

2.5   Method of Analysis 43

2.6   Applications of Complexation.. 45

       2.6.1   Partition Coefficients 46

Chapter 3

Chemical Kinetics

3.1   Chemical Kinetics 48

       3.1.1   Rates and Orders of Reactions 48

       3.1.2   Molecularity 49

       3.1.3   Specific Rate Constants 50

       3.1.4   Units of Basic Rate Constant 50

3.2   Zero Order Reactions 51

       3.2.1   Half Life... 51

       3.2.2   Shelf Life 52

       3.2.3   Suspensions, Apparent Zero-Order Kinetics......................... 52

3.3   First Order Reaction 53

       3.3.1   Half Life... 54

3.4   Second Order Reactions 54

3.5   Determination of Order 56

       3.5.1   Substitution Method.. 56

       3.5.2   Graphic Method 56

       3.5.3   Half-Life Method 56

3.6   Complex Reactions.. 57

       3.6.1   Reversible Reactions 57

       3.6.2   Parallel or Side Reactions 58

       3.6.3   Series or Consecutive Reactions 60

3.7   The Steady State Approximation.. 61

       3.7.1   Michaelis – Menten Equation 61

3.8   Influence of Temperature and other Factors on Reaction Rates.................. 63

       3.8.1   Temperature 63

       3.8.2   Classic Collision Theory of Reaction Rates.......................... 63

       3.8.3   Transition State Theory.. 65

       3.8.4   Effect of the Solvent 65

       3.8.5   Influence of Dielectric Constant 65

       3.8.6   Catalysis.. 65

3.9   Pseudo First Order Reaction 66
3.10   Decomposition and Stabilization of Medicinal Agents 67
          3.10.1   Influence of Light in Photodegradation 69
3.11   Accelerated Stability Studies 70

Chapter 4

Interfacial Phenomena

4.1   Adsorption at Solid Interfaces 74
          4.1.1   Adsorption 74
          4.1.2   Solid-Gas Interface 74
          4.1.3   Applications of Isotherms 80
          4.1.4   The Solid-Liquid Interface 80
          4.1.5   Electric Properties of Interfaces 81
          4.1.6   The Electric Double Layer 81
          4.1.7   Nernst and Zeta Potentials 82
          4.1.8   Wetting Agent 83
          4.1.9   Contact Angle 83
          4.1.10   Applications of Surfactants 85
          4.1.11   Rat-gat Perfusion Technique 86

Chapter 5

Colloids and Macromolecular Systems

5.1   Introduction 87
          5.1.1   Definition 87
5.2   Classification of Colloids 88
          5.2.1   Lyophilic Colloids 89
          5.2.2   Lyophobic Colloids 89
5.3   Dispersion Methods 89
5.4   Purification of Colloids 90
          5.4.1   Dialysis 90
          5.4.2   Electro Dialysis 90
          5.4.3   Ultrafiltration 90
          5.4.3   Association Colloids 91

5.5 Properties of Colloids 93

    5.5.1 Optical Properties 93

    5.5.2 Kinetic Properties of Colloids 96

    5.5.3 Electrical Properties 102

5.6 Solubilisation 105

    5.6.1 Factors Affecting Solubilization 106

Chapter 6

Micromeritics

6.1 Introduction 108

    6.1.1 Significance of Particle size in various Dosage Forms 108

    6.1.2 Significance of Particle Surface Area 108

    6.1.3 Particle and Size Distribution 109

    6.1.4 Particle-Size Distribution 110

    6.1.5 Number and Weight Distribution 110

6.2 Methods for Determining Particle Size 112

    6.2.1 Optical Microscopy 112

    6.2.2 Sieving 113

    6.2.3 Sedimentation Method 113

    6.2.4 Particle Volume Measurement 115

6.3 Particle Shape and Surface Area 116

    6.3.1 Particle Shape 116

    6.3.2 Methods for Determining Surface Area 117

6.4 Derived Properties of Powders 118

    6.4.1 Porosity 118

    6.4.2 Packing Arrangements 119

    6.4.3 Bulkiness 120

    6.4.4 Angle of Repose 120

Chapter 7

Rheology

7.1 Introduction 121

    7.1.1 Importance 121

    7.1.2 Classification 122

7.2   Newtonian System/Fluids 122

    7.2.1   Newton's Law of Flow 122

    7.2.2   Temperature Dependence and Theory of Viscosity 125

7.3   Non–Newtonian Systems 126

    7.3.1   Plastic Flow 126

    7.3.2   Pseudo Plastic Flow 127

    7.3.3   Dilatant Flow – Shear Thickening Systems 128

7.4   Thixotropy 129

    7.4.1   Measurement of Thixotropy 130

    7.4.2   Bulges and Spurs 132

    7.4.3   Negative Thixotropy/Anti Thixotropy 132

7.5   Determination of Rheological Properties 135

    7.5.1   Choice of Viscometer 135

    7.5.2   Types of Rheological Instruments 135

    7.5.3   Principle Methods for Measuring Viscosity 136

    7.5.4   Capillary Viscometer/Ostwald's Viscometer 136

    7.5.5   Falling Sphere Viscometer 139

    7.5.6   Rotational Viscometers 140

    7.5.7   Cop and Bob Viscometer 140

    7.5.8   Cone and Plate Viscometer 143

    7.5.9   Visco Elastic Materials 146

    7.5.10   Pharmaceutical Areas in which Rheology is significant 146

7.6   Rheology of Suspensions 147

    7.6.1   Deflocculated Particles in Newtonian Vehicles 148

    7.6.2   Deflocculated Particles in Non-Newtonian Particles 148

    7.6.3   Flocculated Particles in Newtonian Vehicles 148

    7.6.4   Flocculated Particles in Non-Newtonian Vehicles 148

7.7   Rheology of Emulsions 148

Chapter 8

Dispersed Systems

8.1   Suspensions 152

8.2   Interfacial Properties of Suspended Particles 152

8.3 Theory of Sedimentation 154

    8.3.1 Effect of Brownian Movement 155

    8.3.2 Sedimentation Parameters... 155

    8.3.3 Sedimentation behaviour of Flocculated and Deflocculated Suspensions 157

8.4 Formulation of Suspension.. 159

    8.4.1 Wetting Agents 159

    8.4.2 Deflocculants and Dispersing Agents 160

    8.4.3 Flocculating Agents 160

    8.4.4 Thickness, Protective Colloids and Suspending Agents 160

8.5 Emulsions 161

    8.5.1 Definition of Emulsions 161

8.6 Types of Emulsions 161

    8.6.1 O/W Emulsions 162

    8.6.2 W/O Emulsions 162

    8.6.3 Multiple Emulsions 163

    8.6.4 Micro Emulsions 163

8.7 Identification of Emulsions 163

8.8 Formulation of Emulsions 164

    8.8.1 Raw Materials 165

    8.8.2 Emulsifying Agents 165

    8.8.3 Buffers.. 171

    8.8.4 Density Modifiers 171

    8.8.4 Humectants 172

    8.8.5 Antioxidants... 172

    8.8.6 Preservatives.. 172

    8.8.7 Flavours, Colours and Sweetening Agents 173

8.9 Physical Insolubility of Emulsions 173

    8.9.1 Creaming.. 174

    8.9.2 Flocculation... 174

    8.9.3 Coalescence... 175

    8.9.4 Breaking... 175

    8.9.5 Phase Inversion 176

8.10   Stress Conditions for Evaluating Stability of Emulsions 176

    8.10.1   Aging and Temperature 176

    8.10.2   Centrifugation 177

    8.10.3   Agitation 177

    8.10.4   Phase Separation 178

    8.10.5   Electrophoretic Parameters/Properties 178

8.11   Evaluation and Testing for Emulsions 178

    8.11.1   Methods of Assessing Stability 178

8.12   Theories of Emulsification 179

    8.12.1   Droplet Stabilisation 180

8.13   Chemical Instability of Emulsions 183

8.14   Release of Drugs from Emulsion Formulations 184

CHAPTER 1A

SOLUBILITY

1A.1 Introduction

Solutions are used in pharmaceutical practice and development frequently either as dosage form or for clinical trials material and also the drugs function in solution form in the body. Hence an understanding of properties of solutions and factors that affect solubility is essential to pharmacists for choosing best solvent medium for a drug or combination of drugs.

1A.1.1 Definition of Terms

Solubility can be defined as the ability of the solute to dissolve in a given solvent.

Solution is a homogenous mixture of one or more substances dispersed molecularly in a sufficient quantity of dissolving media. Solution contains two components – solute and solvent. Solute is the substance that is being dissolved and is usually present in smaller proportion. Solvent is the substance that is capable of dissolving solute and usually constitutes the greater proportion in a solution.

A true solution is a homogenous mixture of two or more components in which solute molecules are dispersed as small molecules or ions throughout the solvent. It thus differs from colloidal dispersion where dispersed state molecules or ions are larger.

A saturated solution refers to a solution in which solute is in equilibrium with solid phase at a definite temperature. An unsaturated solution contains solute proportion in lower amounts that is necessary to maintain saturation at definite temperature. Supersaturated solution contains solute in higher proportion that is necessary to maintain saturation at definite temperature.

1A.1.2 Methods of Expressing Solubility

Substance solubility can be expressed in number of parts of solvent required for dissolving one part of solute.

S. No.	Solubility Characteristics	Parts of Solvent Required
1.	Very soluble	Less than 1 part
2.	Freely soluble	1 to 10 parts
3.	Soluble	10 to 30 parts
4.	Sparingly soluble	30 to 100 parts
5.	Slightly soluble	100 to 1000 parts
6.	Very slightly soluble	1000 to 10000 parts
7.	Practically insoluble or insoluble	More than 10000 parts

1A.2   Solute-Solvent Interactions

Ideal solubility depends on the crystalline structure of the solute and solvent. Solute molecule undergoes dissociation from crystal lattice before it goes into solution. This dissociation is accompanied by free energy change. The higher the energy required for dissociation lower the solubility.

Polarity of the solvent contributes to the solubility of the solute. Based on the polarity solvents are of three types:

1. Polar solvents
2. Non polar solvents
3. Semi polar solvents

1A.2.1 Polar Solvents

These solvents dissolve ionic solutes and other polar substances. Factors such as dipole moment, ability of solute to form hydrogen bonds contribute to the polarity of solvents.

Example

Water dissolves aldehydes, ketones, alcohols, phenols etc.

Alcohol with water

In addition, ratio of polar to non polar groups of the molecule also determines solubility character. As the length of a non polar chain of an aliphatic alcohol increases, the solubility in water decreases.

Water solubility increases:

1. If compound contains additional polar groups.

    E.g.: Glycerine

2. Branching of carbon side chain. This is because as branching occurs non polar character decreases and solubility in water increases.

Reasons for high Solubility Character of Polar Solvents

1. High dielectric constant which reduces the force of attraction between oppositely charged ions in the crystal.
2. Ability to break covalent bonds of potentially strong electrolytes.
3. Capability to solvate molecules and ions through dipole interaction forces, which leads to solubility of the compound.

1A.2.2   Non Polar Solvents

These solvents dissolve non polar solutes having same internal pressures.

These can dissolve solutes through induced dipole attractions.

E.g: Dissolution of alkaloidal bases in non polar solvents such as benzene, mineral oil.

They have the poor capacity of solubilizing ionic and polar solutes due to following reasons:

1. Have low dielectric constant
2. Do not form hydrogen bonds
3. Do not break covalent bridges

1A.2.3   Semi Polar Solvents

These solvents induce polarity in non polar substances to certain extent.

E.g.: Propylene glycol increases solubility of water and peppermint oil.

These solvents act as intermediates to increase the solubility of polar and non polar substances.

1A.3   Ideal and Real Solutions

In ideal solutions, all the intermolecular forces such as solvent-solvent, solute-solvent and solute-solute are similar in strength. No heat is evolved or absorbed during the mixing process.

Total vapour pressure of binary system can be measured using equation,

$$P = p_A + p_B \qquad\qquad .....(1A.1)$$

where P is total vapour pressure of system and p_A, p_B are the partial vapour pressures exerted by solute and the solvent.

Vapour pressure of solution is an important property that defines escaping tendency.

Raoult's law states that in an ideal solution, the partial vapour pressure of each volatile constituent is equal to the product of vapour pressure of pure constituent and its mole fraction in the solution.

$$p_A = p_A^o X_A \qquad\qquad .....(1A.2)$$
$$p_B = p_B^o X_B \qquad\qquad .....(1A.3)$$

where p_A, p_B are the partial vapour pressures of the constituents of solution, p_A^o, p_B^o are the vapour pressures of pure components and X_A, X_B are the mole fractions of the constituents.

In an ideal solution where two liquids are mixed together, the vapour pressure of one of the component gets reduced by another and it depends on the mole fraction of the constituents.

Vapour pressure - composition curve for binary system benzene and ethylene chloride is given in Fig. 1A.1 at 50 °C.

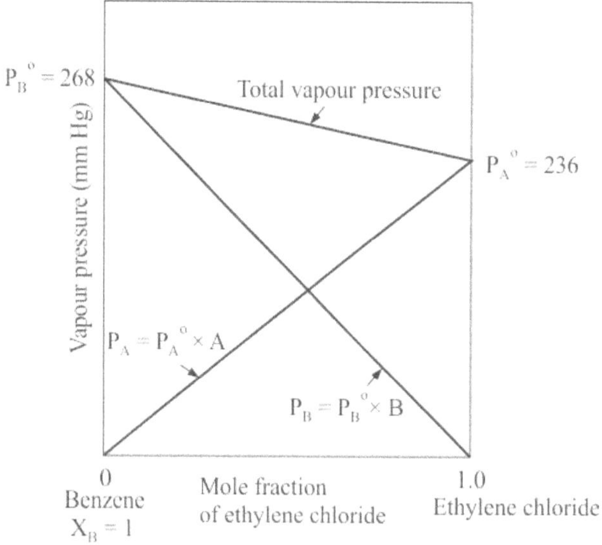

Fig. 1A.1 Vapour pressure composition for an ideal binary system.

Real or non-ideal solutions do not have equal forces of interaction between solute-solute, solute-solvent and solvent-solvent systems.

Heat is either evolved or absorbed when non-ideal solutions are mixed.

These solutions deviate from the Raoult's law. Partial vapour pressure exerted is given by expression

$$P = p^* a \qquad\qquad .....(1A.4)$$

where p^* is the partial pressure exerted by pure component and it refers to thermodynamic activity usually referred to as activity.

When adhesive attractions between molecules of different species are less than cohesive attractions then activities are greater than mole fractions and Raoult's law show positive deviation.

Examples are benzene and ethyl alcohol, chloroform and ethyl alcohol.

Vapour pressure of system showing positive deviation is given in Fig. 1A.2.

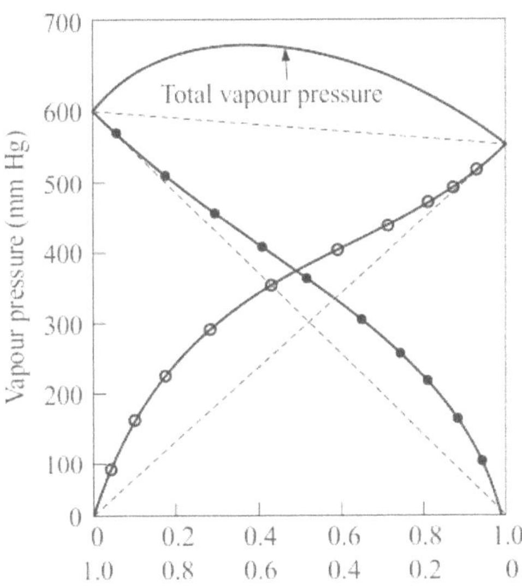

Fig. 1A.2 Vapour pressure of a system showing positive deviation from Raoult's law.

When adhesive forces between different species molecules exceed cohesive forces then Raoult's law shows negative deviation.

Example: Chloroform and acetone.

Vapour pressure of system showing negative deviation is given in Fig. 1A.3.

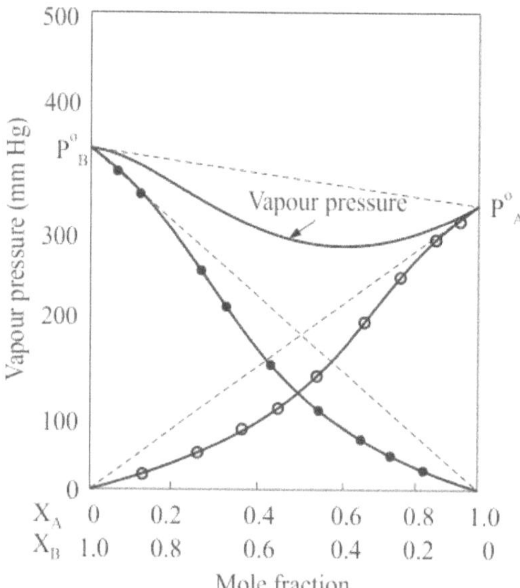

Fig. 1A.3 Vapour pressure of a system showing negative deviation from Raoult's law.

1A.4   Solubility of Gases in Liquids

Solubility of gas in liquid is defined as process of attaining equilibrium between the dissolved gas and the pure gas above the solution.

E.g.: Ammonia water, Hydrochloric acid.

1A.4.1   Factors Affecting Solubility of Gases in Liquids

The following are the factors which affect solubility of gases in liquids:

1. Pressure
2. Temperature
3. Presence of salts
4. Chemical reaction

Pressure

Effect of pressure on solubility of gas in liquids is expressed by Henry's law. This law states that in a very dilute solution at constant temperature the concentration of dissolved gas is proportional to partial pressure of gas above the solution at equilibrium. It is given by expression

$$C = \sigma P$$

$$\ldots\ldots(1A.5)$$

where C refers to the concentration of dissolved gas in grams/litre of solvent, P is partial pressure is millilitres, σ is inverse of Henry's law constant, K or solubility coefficient.

Henry's law relays upon the fact that solubility of gas increases directly with pressure on the gas and may also decrease if pressure above solution is released.

Temperature

As temperature increases, ability of gas to expand also increases and this results in the reduction of solubility of gas in liquids. Hence precautions have to be taken while opening containers of gaseous solutions at elevated temperatures.

Presence of Salts

Gases get liberated upon introduction of either electrolytes or rarely non electrolytes. This is because their occurrence increases in attraction of salt ions or highly polar non electrolytes with liquids. This results in decrease of density of solvent molecules around gaseous molecules and gaseous molecules can easily escape out.

Chemical Reaction

Gases, such as ammonia, hydrogen chloride due to their chemical reaction with water show increase in solubility.

E.g.: Hydrogen chloride is more soluble in water than in oxygen.

Solubility of gases in liquids is expressed using Henry's law constant K, Bunsen absorption coefficient, α.

Henry's law constant K is given by

$$K = \frac{P}{X} \qquad\qquad .....(1A.6)$$

where P is pressure of gas in torrs or atmospheres and X is mole fraction of gas in solution.

$$K = \frac{P}{C \text{ or } M} \qquad\qquad .....(1A.7)$$

where M refers to molality or molarity and C refers to g/l of gas in solution.

1A.5   Solubility of Liquids in Liquids

Frequent mixing of two or more liquids occurs in formulation of many pharmaceutical preparations such as spirits, aromatic waters, elixirs etc. When two liquids are mixed together they exhibit either complete miscibility or partial miscibility.

Complete miscibility is expressed between similar solvents, i.e., in between polar and semi-polar solvents such as water and alcohol, glycerine and alcohol and in between non polar solvents such as benzene and carbon tetrachloride. Partial miscibility is expressed between compounds such as phenol and water, water and ether.

1A.5.1 Factors Affecting Solubility of Liquids in Liquids

The following are the factors affecting solubility of liquids in liquids:

1. Temperature
2. Presence of foreign substances
3. Three component system
4. Dielectric constant
5. Molecular connectivity
6. Molecular surface area

Temperature

Effect of temperature is more on the partially miscible liquids. Mutual solubilities of two conjugate phases may increase when temperature is either increased or decreased.

In case of phenol and water, mutual solubilities of two conjugate systems increases with temperature till a critical solution temperature or upper consolute temperature is attained.

In case of certain liquid pairs, miscibility increased when temperature is lowered and at lower consolute temperature exhibit maximum miscibility.

Mixtures such as nicotine and water exhibit both upper and lower consolute temperature, and ethyl ether and water exhibit neither upper or lower consolute temperature.

Presence of Foreign Substances

The addition of substance to binary system produces ternary system. Its effect on solubility depends on its solubility parameter.

If added substance is soluble in only one of the components of binary system, then the mutual solubility of liquid pair decreases. In this case upper consolute temperature is raised or lower consolute temperature is lowered.

E.g.: If 0.1M naphthalene is added to mixture of phenol and water upper consolute temperature is raised by 20 °C.

If added substance is soluble in both the components of binary system then mutual solubility of liquid pair increase. In this case upper consolute temperature is lowered or lower temperature is raised.

E.g.: Addition of sodium oleate to phenol-water system lowers upper consolute temperature.

This type of increasing mutual solubility is referred to as blending. If added substance is surfactant micellar solubilization phenomenon commences.

Three Component System

Phase equilibria that exist in three component system is usually complex. They are useful in several areas of pharmaceutical processing such as crystallization, salt form selection, etc. A triangular diagram showing solubility of peppermint oil in various proportions of water and polyethylene glycol is given in Fig. 1A.4.

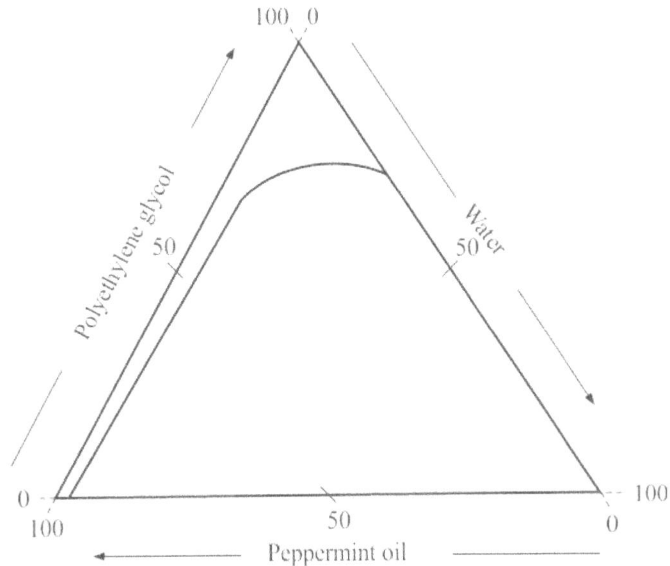

Fig. 1A.4 Triangular diagram showing solubility of peppermint oil in various proportions of water and polyethylene glycol.

Dielectric Constant

As dielectric constant shows considerable effect on the polarity, it is an important factor to be considered in solubility of liquids in liquids. A linear relationship exists when log mole fraction of solute methyl salicylate is plotted against dielectric constant of isopropanol-water mixtures as depicted in Fig. 1A.5.

Molecular Connectivity

Solubility depends on the structural features and functional groups of a particular component. Kier and Hall used molecular connectivity phenomenon to describe solubility. They used structural index χ (chi).

χ term obtained by summing bonds weighted by reciprocal square root number of each bond.

E.g.: Consider propane structure

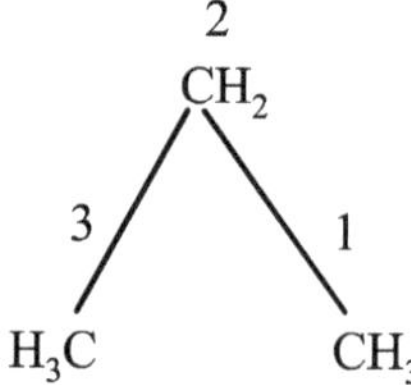

C_1 connected to C_2 by single bond and

C_2 connected to C_3 and C_1 by 2 bonds.

Reciprocal square root valence $= (1.2)^{-1/2} = 0.707$

$$\chi = 0.707 + 0.707 = 1.414$$

Molal solubilities of alcohol, esters in water is correlated using regression analysis.

$$ln\ S = -1.505 - 2.533\,\chi \qquad\qquad .....(1A.8)$$

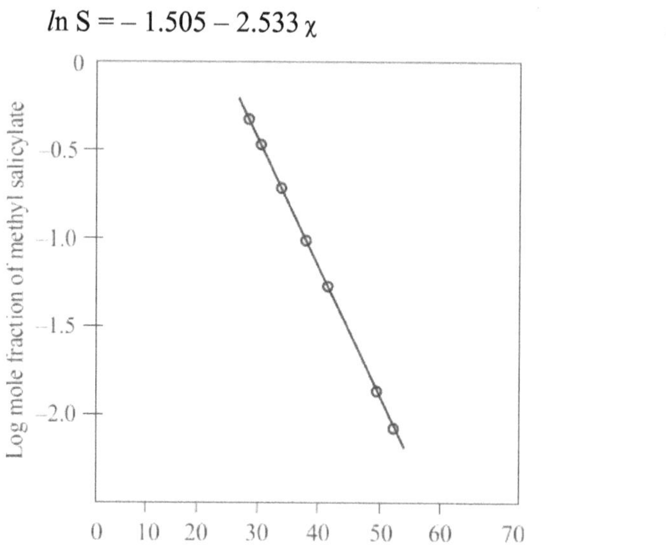

Fig. 1A.5 Solubility of methyl salicylate in isopropanol-water blends of differing dielectric constants.

Molecular Surface Area

Using regression analysis log (solubility) of solute is correlated to its total surface area (TSA)

$$\log (\text{solubility}) = 0.0168 \ (\text{TSA}) + 4.44 \qquad \dots\dots(1A.9)$$

Total surface area includes hydrocarbon (HYSA) and functional surface area (FGSA).

Hence above equation is modified as

$$\text{In (solubility)} = -0.0430 \ (\text{HYSA}) - 0.0586 \ (\text{FGSA}) + 8.003 \ \text{I} + 4.420 \dots\dots(1A.10)$$

where I is indicator variable, HYSA is hydrocarbon surface area and FGSA is functional group surface area.

1A.6   Solubility of Solids in Liquids

Solutions of solids in liquids are most common type of systems in pharmaceutical practice.

1A.6.1   Solubility of Solids in Liquids Determination

A saturated solution is obtained either by stirring excess powdered solute with solvent for several hours at required temperature until equilibrium has been attained or by warming the solvent with excess of solute and allowing the mixture to cool to the required temperature. A sample of saturated solution is obtained for analysis by separating undissolved solid from solution. Filtration is usually used.

To determine solubility of solid in liquid, the solute and solvent must be pure, temperature must be adequately controlled, method of analysing must be reliable and method of separating a sample of saturated solution from undissolved solute must be satisfactory.

Solubility of solute/solid in a liquid for an ideal solution is given by

$$-\log S_2 = \frac{\Delta H_f}{2.303 \, R} \left(\frac{T_0 - T}{TT_0} \right) \qquad \dots\dots(1A.11)$$

where S refers to ideal solubility of solute, T_0 is melting point in absolute degrees, T is absolute temperature of solution, ΔH_f is heat of fusion, R is gas constant.

For non ideal solutions, the activity of solute in a solution is expressed as product of mole fraction and activity coefficient

$$a = S\gamma \qquad \dots\dots(1A.12)$$

where γ is mole fraction scale known as rational activity coefficient.

By applying logarithm to eq. 1A.12

$$\log a = \log S + \log \gamma \qquad .....(1A.13)$$

For ideal solution a = mole fraction, $\gamma = 1$

then

$$-\log a = -\log S = \frac{\Delta H_f}{2.303\, RT}\left(\frac{T_0 - T}{T_0}\right) \qquad .....(1A.14)$$

Therefore by combining equations 1A.13, 1A.14, we get

$$-\log S = \frac{\Delta H_f}{2.303\, R}\left(\frac{T_0 - T}{T_0 T}\right) + \log \gamma \qquad .....(1A.15)$$

$\log \gamma$ value refers to the amount of work carried out in removing the solute molecule and placing it in solvent. It involves three steps:

First step involves removal of molecule from solute phase at definite temperature. The gain in potential energy for process is W_{22}.

Second step involves creation of space in the solvent system for the solute molecule. Work required here is W_{11}.

Third step involves placing solute molecule in solvent system. Decrease in potential energy here is $-W_{12}$.

$$\text{Total work} = W_{22} + W_{11} - W_{12} \qquad .....(1A.16)$$

Logarithm of activity coefficient is given by

$$\ln \gamma = (W_{22} + W_{11} - 2W_{12})\frac{V_2\, \phi_1^2}{RT} \qquad .....(1A.17)$$

where V_2 is molar volume or volume per mole of liquid solute and ϕ_1 is volume fraction, R is gas constant, T is absolute temperature.

As Van der Walls force and follow geometric mean rule,

$$W_{12} = \sqrt{W_{11}\, W_{12}} \qquad .....(1A.18)$$

By substituting eqs. 1A.18 in 1A.17 it becomes

$$\ln \gamma = [W_{11} - 2(W_{11}\, W_{12})^{1/2} + W_{22}]\,\frac{V_2\, \phi_1^2}{RT} \qquad .....(1A.19)$$

Above equation is modified as

$$ln\ \gamma = [(W_{11})^{1/2} - (W_{22})^{1/2}]^2\ \frac{V_2\ \phi_1^2}{RT} \qquad .....(1A.20)$$

$(W)^{1/2}$ terms are solubility parameters and can be designed as δ.

Therefore equation (1A.20) becomes

$$ln\ \gamma = [\delta_1 - \delta_2]\frac{V_2\ \phi_1^2}{RT} \qquad .....(1A.21)$$

When equation (1A.21) is substituted in (1A.15) it is modified as

$$-\log S = \frac{\Delta H_f}{2.303\ RT}\left(\frac{T_0 - T}{T_0}\right) + \frac{V_2\ \phi_1^2}{2.303\ RT}\ [\delta_1 - \delta_2]^2 .....(1A.22)$$

Solubility parameter δ is given by the expression

$$\delta = \left(\frac{\Delta H_v - RT}{V_L}\right)^{1/2} \qquad .....(1A.23)$$

1A.6.2 Factors Affecting Solubility of Solids in Liquids

The following are the factors affecting solubility of solids in liquids:

1. Temperature
2. Nature of solvent, cosolvents
3. Molecular structure of solute
4. pH
5. Particle size of solid
6. Influence of surfactants
7. Effect of complexation

Temperature

Dissolution process is usually an endothermic process i.e., heat is absorbed when dissolution occurs. However they are exceptions where dissolution process is exothermic.

When solubility is plotted against temperature we obtain solubility curves.

Solubility curve is given in Fig. 1A.6

Sodium sulphate exists as decahydrate up to 32.5 $^{\circ}$C and dissolution is endothermic.

After 32.5 °C the process is exothermic as it becomes anhydrous.

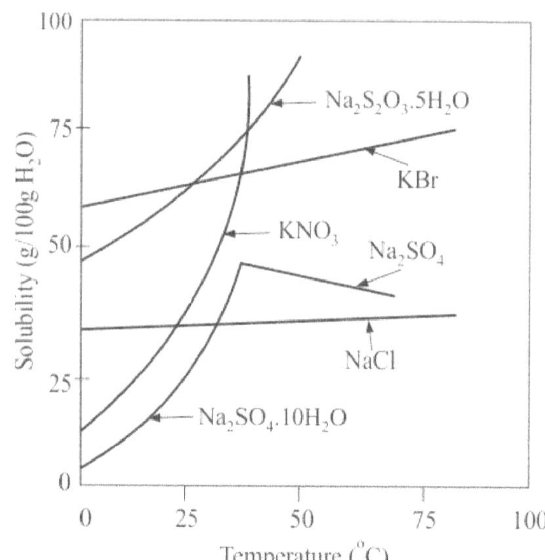

Fig. 1A.6 Influence of temperature on solubility of various salts.

Nature of Solvent, Cosolvents

The importance of statement "Like dissolves Like" applies here. For example polar solvents dissolve polar solutes. In pharmaceutical practice cosolvents such as ethanol or propylene glycol which are miscible with water are used to dissolve solutes in excess of their solubilities.

Molecular Structure of Solute

Even a small change in the molecular structure of compound shows remarkable effect in the solubility.

For example introduction of hydrophilic hydroxyl group can produce a large improvement in water solubility.

pH

Solubility of ionised solutes and pH is extremely important with regard to ionization of weakly acidic and basic drugs as they pass through gastrointestinal track. pH effects degree of ionisation of drug molecule which in turn influences solubility.

Relationship between pH, pKa and solubility is given by Henderson-Hasselbalch equation.

For weakly acidic drug, equation is

$$pH = pKa + \log \frac{[Salt]}{[Acid]} \qquad \ldots\ldots(1A.24)$$

For weakly basic drug,

$$pH = pKw - pKb + \log \frac{[Base]}{[Salt]} \qquad \ldots\ldots(1A.25)$$

Particle Size of Solid

Solubility increases with a decrease in particle size. But too small size causes decrease in solubility.

Changes in interfacial free energy that accompany the dissolution of particles of varying size causes the solubility of a substance to increase with decreasing particle size.

This is indicated by following equation

$$\log \frac{S}{S_0} = \frac{2\gamma M}{2.303\,RT\,Pr} \qquad \ldots\ldots(1A.26)$$

Influence of Surfactants

Weakly acidic drugs and basic drugs are made solubilised by use of surface active agents. Total solubility of acidic drug is expressed as sum of concentration of species in solution

$$D_T = (D) + (D^-) + [D] + [D^-] \qquad \ldots\ldots(1A.27)$$

where (D), (D^-) are non ionized and ionized acid, respectively not in the micelles and $[D]$, $[D^-]$ are non ionized and ionized acid respectively in the micelles.

Partition is express as

For non ionized acid $\quad k^1 = \dfrac{[D]_0}{(D)_0} \qquad \ldots\ldots(1A.28)$

For ionized acid $\quad\quad k^{11} = \dfrac{[D^-]_0}{(D^-)_0} \qquad \ldots\ldots(1A.29)$

In terms of total volume, eq. (1A.28), (1A.29) become

$$k^1 = \frac{[D]\,[1-(M)]}{(D)\,(M)}\,\frac{n!}{r!(n-r)!} \qquad \ldots\ldots(1A.30)$$

$$k^{11} = \frac{[D^-]\,[1-(M)]}{(D^-)\,(M)} \qquad \qquad .....(1A.31)$$

The concentration term, (M) is the volume fraction of surfactant as micelles in solution, amount in true solution is small. Hence $(1 - M)$ is neglected.

Then eq. (1A.30), (1A.31) become

$$[D] = k^1\,(D)\,(M) \qquad \qquad .....(1A.32)$$

$$[D^-] = k^{11}\,(D^-)\,(M) \qquad \qquad .....(1A.33)$$

Total drug solubility, D_T^* in a solution at definite pH in absence of surfactant is given by

$$D_T^* = (D) + (D^-) \qquad \qquad .....(1A.34)$$

For ionized drug is aqueous phase

$$\frac{(D)}{D_T^*} = \frac{(H^+)}{ka + (H^+)} \qquad \qquad .....(1A.35)$$

or

$$D_T^* = (D)\,\frac{ka + (H^+)}{(H^+)} \qquad \qquad .....(1A.36)$$

$$\frac{D_T}{D_T^*} = 1 + (M)\left[\frac{(H^+)\,k^1 + ka\,k^{11}}{ka + (H^+)}\right] \qquad \qquad .....(1A.37)$$

Complexation

When several drugs together with additives interact in solution to form insoluble complexes, apparent solubility of the solute may be increased or decreased due to complex formed.

1A.7   Solubility of Strong Electrolytes

Dissolution process can be exothermic or endothermic process. According to Le Chatelier principle, system tends to adjust in a manner so as to counteract a stress such as increase or decrease in temperature.

Sodium sulphate solubility varies with temperature which is explained in Fig. 1A.6.

Solubility can be explained by means of heat of solution, ΔH. ΔH is known as partial or differential heat of solution which is heat absorbed per mole when a small quantity of solute is added to large quantity of solution. Total or Integral heat of solution is heat absorbed when one mole of solute is dissolved in enough solvent to produce solution of specified concentration.

Heat of solution of crystalline substance is the sum of heat of sublimation of solid and heat of hydration of ions in solution

$$\Delta H \text{ (solution)} = \Delta H_{subl} + \Delta H_{hyd} \qquad .....(1A.38)$$

where ΔH_{sub} – Heat of sublimation

$\qquad \Delta H_{hyd}$ – Heat of hydration

Heat of sublimation is the energy required to separate one mole of crystal into its ions in gaseous state or to vapourise solid.

$$NaCl_{solid} \longrightarrow Na^+_{gas} + Cl^-_{gas}$$

Heat of hydration is the heat liberated when gaseous ions are hydrated.

$$Na^+_{gas} + Cl^-_{gas} \xrightarrow{\ H_2O\ } Na^+_{aq} + Cl^-_{aq}$$

In ideal solution $\Delta H_{hyd} = 0$ as heat absorbed is only that required to transform crystals to liquid state.

1A.8   Solubility of Slightly Soluble Electrolytes

Solubility product k_{sp} is used to describe the process of dissolution of slightly soluble electrolytes to form saturated solutions.

Example for slightly soluble electrolyte is silver chloride when excess solid in equilibrium with ions in saturated solution at specific temperature is represented as

$$AgCl_{solid} \rightleftharpoons Ag^+ + Cl^- \qquad .....(1A.39)$$

Equilibrium expression for it is,

$$k = \frac{[Ag^+][Cl^-]}{[AgCl_{solid}]} \qquad .....(1A.40)$$

As concentration of solid phase is constant

$$k_{sp} = [Ag^+] [Cl^-] \qquad .....(1A.41)$$

If an ion in common either Ag^+ or Cl^- is added then equilibrium is altered.

For example addition of sodium chloride increases chloride ion concentration and

$$[Ag^+] [Cl^-] > k_{sp}$$

Some of AgCl precipitates until equilibrium is attained. Hence addition of common ion reduces the solubility of slightly soluble electrolytes.

Salts having no ion in common with slightly soluble electrolyte if added at modulate concentration causes increase in the solubility because of reduction of activity coefficient.

$$k_{sp} = a_{Ag^+} + a_{Cl} \qquad\qquad .....(1A.42)$$

Because activities can be replaced by product of concentration and activity coefficients,

$$k_{sp} = \left[Ag^+\right]\left[Cl^-\right]\gamma_{Ag^+} + \gamma_{Cl^-} = \left[Ag^+\right]\left[Cl^-\right]\gamma_\pm^2$$

$$\frac{k_{sp}}{\gamma_\pm^2} = [Ag^+][Cl^-]$$

and
$$\text{solubility} = [Ag^+] = [Cl^-] = \frac{\sqrt{k_{sp}}}{\gamma_\pm} \qquad\qquad .....(1A.43)$$

1A.9   Solubility of Weak Electrolytes

Most of the drugs are either weakly acidic or weakly basic, which react with strong acids and bases at definite pH range and exists as ions that are ordinarily soluble in water.

Example is carboxylic acids containing more than five carbons react with dilute carbonates and bicarbonates form soluble salts.

Hydroxy acids such as tartaric acid are soluble in water because they are solvated through hydroxyl groups.

Salicylic acid is soluble in alcohol and alkalies. This is because OH group is involved in intermolecular hydrogen bond.

Many compounds containing basic nitrogen atom in the molecule such as sulphonamides are important in pharmacy. These exist as salts.

E.g.: Sulfadiazine sodium

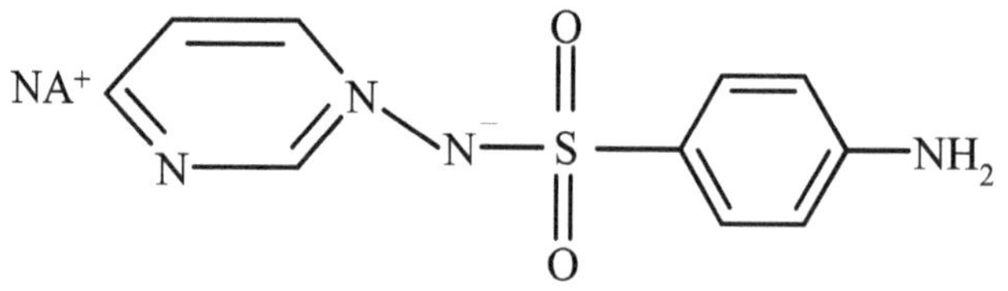

Oxygen of sulfonyl group withdraw electrons from sulphur atom which results in electrons of N : H bond being held more close to nitrogen atom. Hydrogen is less firmly held and can be easily removed.

Solubility of weak electrolytes is greatly influenced by pH.

Consider acid form of drug, HP with soluble ionised form P⁻.

Equilibria in saturated solution can be expressed as

$$HP_{solid} \rightleftharpoons HP_{sol} \qquad\qquad .....(1A.44)$$

$$HP_{sol} + H_2O \rightleftharpoons H_3O^+ + P^- \qquad\qquad .....(1A.45)$$

Equilibrium constant for solution equilibrium is

$$S_o = [HP]_{sol} \qquad\qquad .....(1A.46)$$

Constant for acid-base equilibrium is

$$ka = \frac{[H_3O^+][P^-]}{[HP]} \qquad\qquad .....(1A.47)$$

$$[P^-] = \frac{ka\,[HP]}{[H_3O^+]} \qquad\qquad .....(1A.48)$$

Total solubility constitutes both concentration of undissociated and ionised form

$$S = [HP] + [P^-] \qquad\qquad .....(1A.49)$$

Substituting S_0 from eq. (1A.46) and $[P^-]$ from eq. (1A.48), the eq. (1A.49) becomes

$$S = S_o + ka\,\frac{S_0}{[H_3O^+]} \qquad\qquad .....(1A.50)$$

$$S = S_0 \left(1 + \frac{ka}{[H_3O^+]}\right) \qquad\qquad .....(1A.51)$$

This equation can be modified as

$$(S - S_0) = ka\,\frac{S_0}{[H_3O^+]} \qquad\qquad .....(1A.52)$$

By applying logarithm to eq. (52), it becomes

$$Log\,(S - S_0) = \log ka + \log S_0 - \log [H_3O^+] \qquad\qquad .....(1A.53)$$

and finally

$$pHp = pKa + \log \frac{S - S_0}{S_0}$$

where pHp is pH below which drug separates from solution as undissociated acid.

CHAPTER 1B

DISTRIBUTION PHENOMENA

1B.1   Introduction

Distribution is a reversible process. In general distribution is mainly seen in biological fluids. In this case the rate of exchange between plasma and tissue vary widely depending on the type of tissue and drug partition characteristics. When distribution is rapid, the body behaves kinetically as a single homogeneous pool and the plasma concentration time course may be adequately described by a single exponential. On the other hand the kinetics of drug disposition often exhibit multi exponential characteristics. Each additional exponential has been interpreted to represent a group of tissues requiring progressively more time in which to achieve a steady state in drug distribution.

1B.2   Partition Coefficient

If a substance which is soluble in both components of a mixture of immiscible liquids is dissolved in such a mixture, then equilibrium is attained at constant temperature it is found that the solute is distributed between the two liquids in such a way that the ratio of the activities of the substance in each liquid is a constant. This is known as the 'Nernst distribution law", which can be expressed by equation

$$\frac{a_A}{a_B} = \text{constant} \qquad\qquad .....(1B.1)$$

where a_A and a_B are the activities of the solute in the solvent A and B respectively; when the solution is dilute and when the solute behave ideally, the activities may be replaced by concentration (C_A and C_B)

$$\frac{C_A}{C_B} = k \qquad\qquad .....(1B.2)$$

where the constant k is known as "distribution coefficient or partition coefficient".

In case of sparingly soluble substance, k is approximately equal to the ratio of the solubilities (S_A and S_B) of the solute in each liquid i.e.,

$$\frac{S_A}{S_B} = k \qquad\qquad \text{.....(1B.3)}$$

In most other systems, however, deviation from ideal behaviour invalidates eq. 1B.3. For example, if the solute exists as monomers in solvent A and as dimer in solvent B, the distribution coefficient is given by eq. 1B.4, in which the square root of the concentration of the dimeric form is used.

$$k = \frac{C_A}{\sqrt{C_B}} \qquad\qquad \text{.....(1B.4)}$$

If the dissociation into ions occurs in the aqueous layer, B of a mixture of immiscible liquid, then the degree of dissociation (α) should be taken into account, as indicated by eq. 1B.5.

$$k = \frac{C_A}{C_B(1-\alpha)} \qquad\qquad \text{.....(1B.5)}$$

The solvents in which the concentration of the solute is expressed should be indicated when partition coefficient are quoted. For example, a partition coefficient of 2 for a solute distributed between oil and water may also be expressed as a partition coefficient between water and oil at 0.5. This can be represented as

$$k_{water}^{oil} = 2 \text{ and } k_{oil}^{water} = 0.5.$$

The abbreviation k_w^0 is often used for the former.

1B.2.1 Effect of Partition of Ionic Dissociation and Molecular Association

The solute can exist partly or wholly as associated molecules in one of the phases or it may dissociate into ion in either of the liquid phases. The distribution law applies only to the concentration of the species common to both phases, namely, the monomer as simple molecule of the solute.

Consider the distribution of benzoic acid between an oil phase and a water phase. When it is neither associated in the oil nor dissociated into ion in the water. When association and dissociation occurs, however, the situation becomes more complicated. In general case where benzoic acid associated in the oil phase and dissociates in the aqueous phase in shown in Fig. 1B.1.

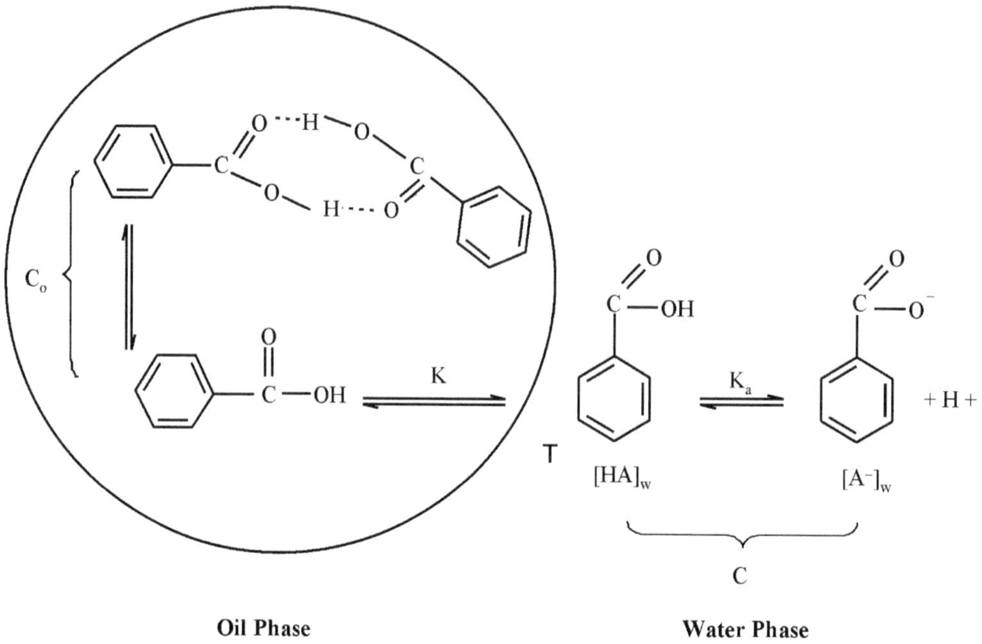

Fig. 1B.1 Schematic representation of distribution of benzoic acid between a water and an oil phase is depicted as a magnified oil droplet in an oil-in water emulsion.

Two cases will be treated. First according to Garrett and Woods benzoic acid is considered to be distributed between the two phases, peanut oil and water. Although benzoic acid undergoes dimerization in many non polar solvents, it does not associate in peanut oil. It ionizes in water to a degree, however, depending on the pH of the solution. Therefore in Fig. 1B.1 for the case under consideration, C_0 the total concentration of benzoic acid in the oil phase is equal to $[HA]_0$, the monomer concentration in the oil phase, because association does not occur in peanut oil.

The species common to both the oil and water phase are the un-associated and un- dissociated benzoic acid molecules. The distribution is expressed as

$$k = \frac{[HA]_0}{[HA]_w} = \frac{C_0}{[HA]_w} \qquad\qquad .....(1B.6)$$

where k is the true distribution coefficient, $[HA]_0 = C_0$ is the molar concentration of the simple benzoic acid molecules in the oil phase and $[HA]_w$ is the molar concentration of the un-dissociated acid in the water phase.

The total acid concentration obtained by analysis of the aqueous phase is

$$C_w = [HA]_w + [A^-]_w \qquad\qquad .....(1B.7)$$

and the experimentally observed or apparent distribution coefficient is

$$k^1 = \frac{[HA]_0}{[HA]_w + [A^-]_w} = \frac{C_0}{C_w} \qquad .....(1B.8)$$

As seen in Fig. 1B.1, the observed distribution coefficient depends on two equilibria; the distribution of the un-dissociated acid between the immiscible phase as expressed in eq. (1B.6) and the species distribution of the acid in the aqueous phase, which depends on the hydrogen ion concentration $[H_3O^+]$ and the dissociation constant k_a of the acid, where

$$k_a = \frac{[H_3O^+][A^-]_w}{[HA]_w} \qquad .....(1B.9)$$

Association of benzoic acid in peanut oil does not occur and k_d (the equilibrium constant for dissociation of associated benzoic acid into monomer in the oil phase) can be neglected in this case.

Given these equations and the fact the concentration of the acid in the aqueous phase before distribution, assuming equal volumes of the two phases,

$$C = C_0 + C_w \qquad .....(1B.10)$$

One arrives at the combine result

$$\frac{k_a + [H_3O^+]}{C_w} = \frac{k_a}{C} = \frac{k+1}{C}[H_3O^+] \qquad .....(1B.11)$$

Eq. 1B.11 is a linear equation of the form $y = a + bx$, and therefore a plot of $[k_a + [H_3O^+]]/C_w$ against $[H_3O^+]$ yields a straight line with a slope $b = (k + 1)/C$ and an intercept $a = k_a/C$. The true distribution coefficient k can thus be obtained over the range of hydrogen ion concentration considered. Alternatively, the true distribution constant could be obtained according to eq. (1B.6) by analysis of the oil phase and of the water phase, at a sufficiently low pH (2) at which the acid would exist completely in the unionized form. One of the advantage of eq. (1B.11), however is the oil phase need be analyzed; only the hydrogen ion concentration and C_w; the total concentration remaining in the aqueous phase at equilibrium need be determined.

Second, let us consider the cane in which the solute is associated in the organic phase and exists as simple molecules in the aqueous phase. If benzoic acid is distributed between benzene and acidified water, it exists mainly as associated molecules in the benzene layer and as un-dissociated molecules in the aqueous layer.

The equilibrium between simple molecules HA and associated molecules $[HA]_n$ in bezene is

$$(HA)_n \rightleftharpoons n\,(HA)$$

Associated molecules   Simple molecules

and the equilibrium constant expressing the dissociation of associated molecules into simple molecules in this solvent is

$$k_d = \frac{[HA]_0^n}{[(HA)_n]} \qquad \qquad .....(1B.12)$$

or

$$[HA]_0 = \sqrt[n]{k_d}\ \sqrt[n]{[(HA)_n]} \qquad \qquad .....(1B.13)$$

Because benzoic acid exists predominantly in the form of double molecules in benzene, C_0 can replace $[(HA)_n]$, where C_0 is the total molar concentration of the solute in the organic layer. The eq. (1B.13) can be written approximately as

$$[HA]_0 \cong constant \times \sqrt{C_0} \qquad \qquad .....(1B.14)$$

In conformity with distribution law as given in eq. (1B.6), the true distribution coefficient is always expressed in terms of simple species common to both phases, i.e., in terms of $[HA]_n$ and $[HA]_0$. In the benzene-water system, $[HA]_0$ is given by eq. (1B.14) and the modified distribution constant becomes

$$k^{11} = \frac{[HA]_0}{[HA]_w} = \frac{\sqrt{C_0}}{[HA]_w} \qquad \qquad .....(1B.15)$$

1B.2.2 Extraction

To determine the efficiency with which one solvent can extract a compound from a second solvent – an operation commonly employed in analytic chemistry and in organic chemistry – we follow glass tone. Suppose that w gram of a solute is extracted repeatedly from v_1 ml of the one solvent with successive partition of v_2 ml of second solvent, which is immiscible with first.

Let w_1 be the weight of the solute remaining in the original solvent after extracting with the first portion of the other solvent. Then the concentration of solute remaining in the first solvent is (w_1/v_1) g/ml and the concentration of the solute in the extracting solvent is $(w_2 - w_1)$ g/ml. The distribution coefficient is thus.

$$k = \frac{\text{Concentration of solute in original solvent}}{\text{Concentration of solute in extracting solvent}}$$

$$k = \frac{w_1/v_1}{\left(w_1 - w_2\right)/v_2} \qquad \qquad .....(1B.16)$$

or

$$w_1 = w \, \frac{kv_1}{kv_1 + v_2} \qquad \qquad .....(1B.17)$$

The process can be repeated and after n extraction

$$w_n = w \left[\frac{kv_1}{kv_1 + v_2} \right]^n \qquad \qquad .....(1B.18)$$

By use of this equation, it can be shown that most efficient extraction results when n is large and v_2 is small, in other words, when a large number of extractions are carried out with small portions of extracting liquid.

1B.3   Solubility and Partition Coefficients

Hansch observed a relationship between aqueous solubilities of non electrolytes and partitioning. Yalkowsky and Valvani obtained an equation for determining the aqueous solubility of liquid or crystalline organic compound.

$$\log s = -\log k - 1.11 \, \frac{\Delta sf \, (mp - 25)}{13\,64} + 0.54 \qquad .....(1B.19)$$

where s is aqueous solubility in moles (lit), k is the octanol water partition coefficient, Δsf is the molar entropy of fusion and mp is the melting point of the solid compound on the centigrade scale. For a liquid compound, mp is assigned a value of 25, so that the second right hand term of eq. (1B.19) becomes zero.

The entropy of fusion and the partition coefficient can be estimated from the chemical structure of the compound. For rigid molecules, $\Delta sf = 13.5$ entropy exists, for molecules with n greater than five non hydrogen atoms in a flexible chain.

$$\Delta sf = 13.5 + 2.5 \, (n - 5) \qquad \qquad .....(1B.20)$$

Leo *et al.,* provided partition coefficient for a large number of compounds. When experimental values are not available, group contribution methods are available for estimating partition coefficient.

1B.3.1 Preservative Action of Weak Acids in Oil-Water Systems

Solution of foods, drugs and cosmetics are subject to deterioration by the enzymes of micro organisms that act as catalyst in decomposition reaction. These enzymes are produced by yeast, moulds and bacteria and such micro organisms must be destroyed or inhibited to prevent deterioration. Sterilization and the addition of preservatives (chemicals) are common methods used in pharmacy to preserve drug solutions against attack by various micro organisms. Benzoic acid in the form of its soluble salt, sodium benzoate is often used for this purpose because it produces no injurious effect in humans when taken internally in small quantities.

Rahn and Conn showed that the preservative or bacteriostatic action of benzoic acid and similar acids is due almost entirely to the un-dissociated acid and not to the ionic form. These investigators found that the yeast *Saccharomyces ellipsoideus*, which grows normally at a pH of 2.5 to 7.0 in the presence of strong inorganic acids or salts, ceased to grow in the presence of un-dissociated benzoic acid when the concentration of the acid reached 25 mg/100 ml. The preservative action of un-dissociated benzoic acid as compared with the ineffectiveness of the benzoic ion is presumably due to the relative ease with which the unionized molecule penetrated living membrane and conversely, the difficulties with which the ion does so. The undissociated molecule, consisting of a large nonpolar portion is soluble in the lipoidal membrane of the micro organism and penetrates rapidly.

Bacteria in oil-water system are generally located in the aqueous phase and at the oil-water interface. Therefore, the efficacy of a weak acid, such as benzoic acid, as a preservative for these systems is largely a result of the concentration of the undissociated acid in the aqueous phase.

To calculate the total concentration of benzoic acid that must be added to preserve an oil-water mixture, we proceed as follows.

Let us take the peanut oil-water mixture considered by Garrett and woods and begin by writing the expression.

$$C = g\, C_0 + C_w = g\, [HA]_0 + [HA]_w + [A^-]_w \qquad .....(1B.21)$$

where $g = v_0/v_w$, the volume ratio of the two phases is needed when the volumes are not equal, C is the original concentration of the acid in the water phase before the aqueous solution is equilibrated with peanut oil, C_0 is the molar concentration of the simple dissociated molecules in the oil, because the acid does not dimerize or dissociate in the organic phase, and C_w the molar concentration of benzoic acid in water is equal to the sum of the two terms $[HA]_w$ and $[A^-]_w$ in this ionizing solvent. It is further assumed that concentrations are approximately equal to activities.

The distribution of total benzoic acid among the various species in this system depends upon the distribution coefficient, k, the dissociation constant, ka, of the acid in the aqueous phase, the phase valence ratio and the hydrogen ion concentration of aqueous phase. To account for the first effect, we introduce the term $k = [HA]_0/[HA]_w$ or $[HA]_0 = k[HA]_w$ into eq. (1B.21). We write the dissociation constant $ka = [H_3O^+] [A^-]_w/[HA]_w$ or the ionic species, $[A^-]_w = ka\,[HA]_w / [H_3O^+]$ to account for the influence of ka and $[H_3O^+]$ and substitute it also into eq. (1B.21). The expression then become

$$C = kg\, [HA]_w + [HA]_w + ka[HA]_w / [H_3O^+] \qquad .....(1B.22)$$

Factoring out $[HA]_w$, we have

$$C = \left(\frac{kg + 1 + ka}{\left[H_3O^+\right]} \right) (HA)_w \qquad \qquad .....(1B.23)$$

or

$$(HA)_w = \frac{C}{\dfrac{kg + 1 + ka}{\left[H_3O^+\right]}} \qquad \qquad .....(1B.24)$$

Eq. (1B.23) and (1B.24) can be used to calculate the concentration C of total acid that must be added to the entire two phase system. To obtain a final specified concentration $[HA]_w$ of undissociated acid in the aqueous phase buffered at a definite pH or hydrogen ion concentration.

Kazmi and Mitchell and Bean *et al.,* proposed calculations for presenting solubilized and emulsified system that are slightly different from the Garrett and Woods.

In case where benzoic acid exists as a dimer in the oil phase, the modified distribution coefficient is k" = $(1/[HA]_w)$ and there from eq. (1B.21) becomes

$$C = k''^2 g \, [HA]_w^2 + [HA]_w + ka[HA]_w \, / \, [H_3O^+] \qquad .....(1B.25)$$

and finally

$$C = k''^2 \, g[HA]_w + 1 + \left(\frac{ka}{[H_3O]} \right) [HA]_w \qquad \qquad .....(1B.26)$$

1B.4   Drug Action and Partition Coefficients

More than 100 years ago Meyer and Overton prepared the hypothesis that the narcotic action of a non specific drug is a function of the distribution coefficient of the compound between a lipoidal medium and water. Later it was concluded that narcosis was a function only of the concentration of the drug in the lipids of the cell. Thus, a wide variety of drugs of different chemical types should produce equal narcotic action at equal concentration in the lipoidal cell substance. Actually, as will be seen shortly, this is a restatement of the theory, first proposed by Ferguson and generally accepted today. The equal degrees of narcotic action should occur at equal thermodynamic activities of the drugs in solution.

The activity of a vapour is obtained approximately by the use of the equation.

$$\frac{p_{nar}}{p^0} = a_{nar} \qquad \qquad .....(1B.27)$$

If p_{nar} is the partial pressure of a narcotic in solution just necessary to bring about narcosis and p^0 is the vapour pressure of the pure liquid, narcosis will occur at a thermodynamic activity of α_{nar}.

FICK'S LAWS OF DIFFUSION

1C.1　Introduction

Diffusion is defined as a process of mass transfer of individual molecules of a substance brought about by random molecular motion and associated with a driving force such as a concentration gradient. The mass transfer of solvent or solute forms the basis for many important phenomena in the pharmaceutical sciences. For example, diffusion of a drug across a biological membrane is required for a drug to be absorbed into and eliminated from the body and even for it to get to the site of action within a particular cell on the negative side. The shelf life of a drug product could be significantly reduced if a container or closure does not prevent solvent or drug loss or if it does not prevent the absorption of water vapour into the container. These and many more important phenomena have a basis in diffusion. Drug release from a variety of drug delivery systems, drug absorption and elimination, dialysis, osmosis and ultra filtration are some of the examples.

1C.1.1　Drug Absorption and Elimination

Diffusion through biologic membranes is an essential step for drugs entering or leaving the body. It is also an important component along with concentration for efficient drug distribution throughout the body and into tissues and organs. Diffusion can occur through the lipoidal bilayer of cells. This is termed transcellular diffusion. On the other hand, paracellular diffusion occurs through the spaces between adjacent cells. In addition to diffusion, drugs and nutrients also traverse biologic membranes using membrane transporters and to a lesser extent, cell surface receptors.

Membrane transporters are specialised proteins that facilitate drug transport across biological membranes. The interaction between drugs and transporters can be classified as energy dependent (i.e., active transport) or energy independent (i.e., facilitated diffusion). Membrane transporters are located in every organ responsible for the absorption, distribution, metabolism and excretion of drug substances.

1C.1.2 Drug Release

Elementary drug release is an important process that literally attends nearly every person in everyday life. Drug release is multistep process that includes diffusion, disintegration, deaggregation and dissolution. These processes are important for the release of drug from formulation. Common examples are the release of steroids such as hydrocortisone from topical over-the-counter creams and ointments for the treatment of skin rashes and the release of acetaminophen from a tablet that is taken by mouth.

1C.1.3 Osmosis

Osmosis was originally defined as the passage of the both solute and solvent across a membrane but now refers to an action in which only the solvent is transferred. The solvent passes through a semi permeable membrane to dilute the solution containing solute and solvent. The passage of solute together with solvent now is called diffusion or dialysis. Osmotic drug release system uses osmotic pressure, as a driving force for the controlled delivery of drugs. A simple osmotic pump consists of an osmotic core (containing drug with or without an osmotic agent) and is coated with a semi permeable membrane. The semi permeable membrane has an orifice for drug release from the "pump". The dosage form after coming in contact with aqueous fluids, imbibes water at a rare determined by the fluid permeability of the membrane and osmotic pressure of core formulation. The osmotic imbibition of water results in high hydrostatic pressure inside the pump, which causes the flow of the drug solutions through the delivery orifice.

1C.1.4 Ultra Filtration and Dialysis

Ultra filtration is used to separate colloidal particles and macromolecules by the use of membrane. Hydraulic pressure is used to force the solvent through membrane, where as the micro porous membrane prevents the passage of molecules. Ultra filtration is similar to a process called reverse osmosis.

Dialysis is a separate process based on unequal rates of passage of solutes and solvents through micro porous membranes.

Haemodialysis is used in treating kidney malfunction to rid the blood of metabolic waste product while preserving the high molecular weight components of blood. In ordinary osmosis and as well as in dialysis, separation is spontaneous and does not involve the high applied pressers of ultra filtration and reverse osmosis.

1C.2 Steady-State Diffusion

1C.2.1 Thermodynamic Basis

Mass transfer is the movement of molecules in response to an applied diving force. Convective and diffusive mass transfers are important to many pharmaceutical science applications. Mass transfer is the kinetic process, occurring in the system that is not in equilibrium. To better understand the thermodynamic basis of mass transfer, consider an isolated system consisting of two sections separated by an imaginary membrane (Fig. 1C.1). At equilibrium, the temperature T, pressure P and chemical potentials μ of each two species A and B are equal in the two sections. In this isolated system is unperturbed, it will remain at this thermodynamic equilibrium indefinitely.

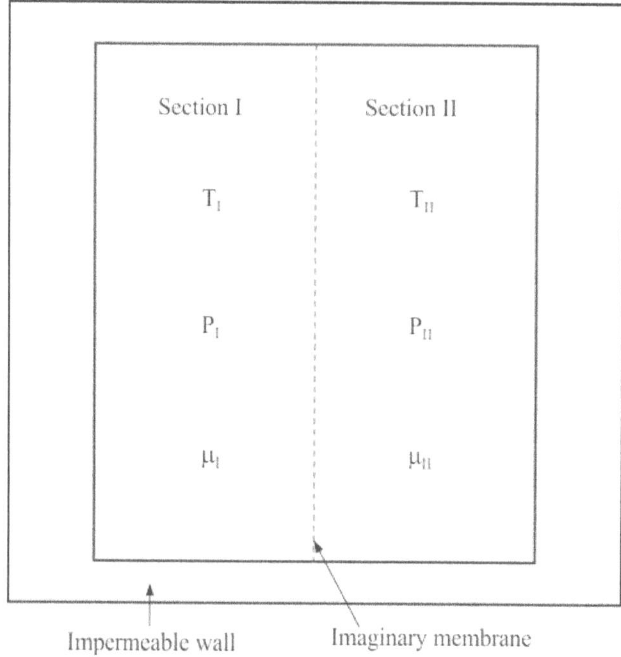

Fig. 1C.1 Isolated system consisting of two sections separated by Imaginary membrane.

Suppose that the chemical potential of one of the species A is now increased in section I so that M_A I > M_A II, because the chemical potential of A is related to its concentration. The ideality of the solution and the temperature, this perturbation of the system can be achieved by increasing the concentration of A in section I. The system will respond to this perturbation by establishing a new thermodynamic equilibrium. Although it could be re establish the equilibrium by altering any of the 3 variables in the system   (T, P or μ).

Let's assume that it will re equilibrate the chemical potential leaving T and P unaffected. If the membrane separating the two sections will allow for the passage of species A, then equilibrium will be re established by the movement of species A from section I to section II until the chemical potentials of section I and II are once again equal. The movement of mass is response to a spatial gradient in chemical potential as a result of random molecular motion (i.e., Brownian motion) is called diffusion.

1C.3   Fick's Laws of Diffusion

1C.3.1   Fick's First Law

The amount M of material flowing through a unit cross section, δ of a barrier in unit time t is known as the flux J

$$J = \frac{dM}{S.dt} \qquad \qquad .....(1C.1)$$

The flux in turn is proportional to the concentration gradient dc/dx

$$J = -D\frac{dc}{dx} \qquad \qquad .....(1C.2)$$

where D is the diffusion coefficient of diffusant in cm^2 /see. C is the concentration in g/cm^3 and x is the distance in cm of movement perpendicular to the surface of the barrier. In eq. (1C.1). The mass M is usually given in grams or moles, the barrier surface area S in cm^2 and the time t in seconds. The unit of J are g/cm^2 sec. The negative sign of eq. (1C.2) signifies that diffusion occur in a direction opposite to that of increasing concentration. That is diffusion occur in the direction of decreasing concentration of diffusant; thus the flux is always a positive quantity. Diffusion will stop when the concentration gradient no longer exists (i.e., when dc/dx = 0).

Although the diffusion coefficient D or diffusivity as it is often called appear to be proportionality constant; it does not ordinarily remain constant. D is affected by concentration, temperature, pressure, solvent properties and the chemical nature of the diffusant. Therefore D is referred to more correctly as diffusion coefficient rather than as a constant. eq. (1C.2) is known as Fick's first law.

1C.3.2   Fick's Second Law

Fick's second law of diffusion forms the basis for most mathematical models of diffusion process. One often wants to examine the rate of change of diffusant concentration at a point in the system. An equation for mass transport that emphasizes the change in concentration with time at a definite location rather than the mass diffusing across a unit area of barrier in unit time is known as Fick's second law. This diffusion equation is derived as follows.

The concentration C, in a particular volume element (Fig. 1C.2 and 1C.3) changes only as a result of net flow of diffusing molecules into or out of the region. A difference in concentration results from a difference in input and output. The concentration of diffusant in the volume element changes with time, that is $\Delta c/\Delta t$, as the flux or amount diffusing changes with distance $\Delta T/\Delta R$ in the x direction, or

$$\frac{\partial c}{\partial t} = -\frac{\partial j}{\partial x} \qquad \qquad .....(1C.3)$$

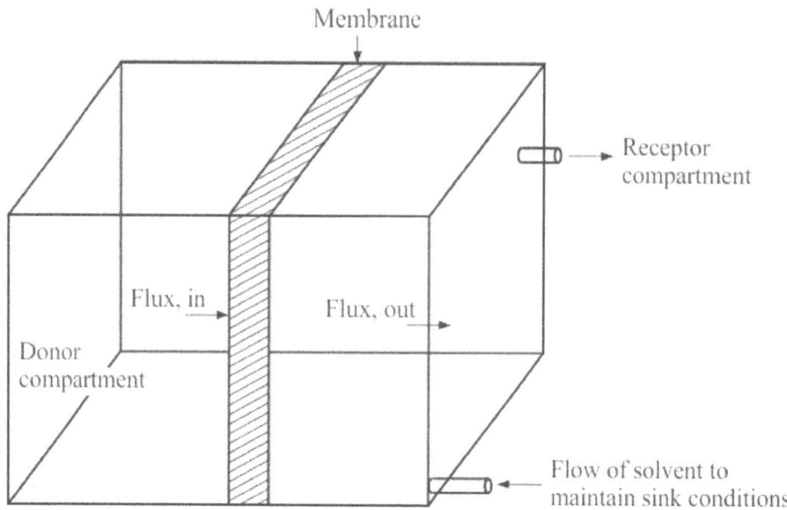

Fig. 1C.2 Diffusion cell. The donor compartment contains diffusant at concentration c.

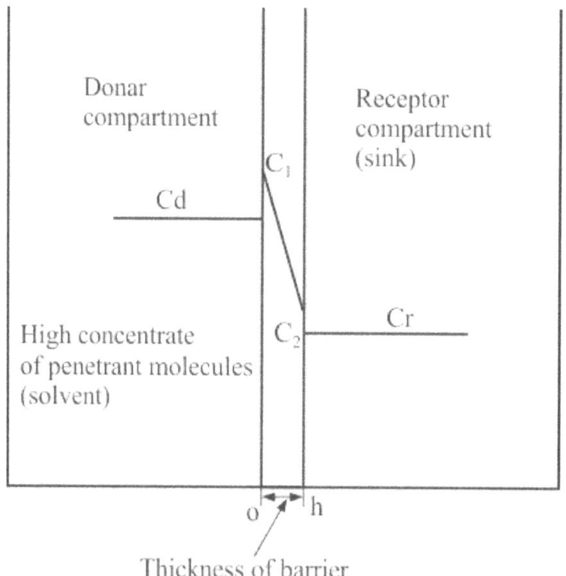

Fig. 1C.3 Concentration gradient of diffusant across the diaphragm of diffusion cell. It is normal for the concentration curve to increase or decrease sharply at the boundaries of barrier because in general, C_1 is different from C_d and C_2 is different from C_r. The concentration C_1 would be equal to C_d for Example, only if $K - C_1/C_d$ had a value of unity.

Differentiating the first law expansion equation (1C.2) with respect to x, one obtain

$$-\frac{\partial j}{\partial x} = D\frac{\partial^2 c}{\partial x^2} \qquad .....(1C.4)$$

Substituting $\partial c / \partial t$ from eq. (1C.3) into eq. (1C.4) results in Fick's second law, namely

$$\frac{\partial c}{\partial x} = D\frac{\partial^2 c}{\partial x^2} \qquad .....(1C.5)$$

Eq. (1C.5) represent diffusion only in the x direction. If one wishes to express concentration changes of diffusant in 3 dimensions, Fick's second law is written in the general form.

$$\frac{\partial c}{\partial x} = D\left[\frac{\partial^2 c}{\partial x^2} + \frac{\partial^2 c}{\partial y^2} + \frac{\partial^2 c}{\partial z^2}\right] \qquad .....(1C.6)$$

This expression is not usually needed in pharmaceutical problems of diffusion, however, because movement in one direction is sufficient to describe most cases. Fick's second law states that the change in concentration with time in a particular region is proportional to the change in the concentration gradient at that point in the system.

CHAPTER 2

COMPLEXATION

2.1 Definition

Complexation is defined as a reversible association of substrate and ligand to form a new species.

2.1.1 Classification of Complexes

The complexes are classified as follows such as

1. *Metal ion complexes*
    - (a)   Inorganic type
    - (b)   Chelates
    - (c)   Olefin type   (d)   Aromatic type

2. *Organic Molecular complexes*
    - (a) Donor-acceptor type
    - (b) Charge transfer type
    - (c)   Drug and caffeine complexes
    - (d)   Polymer type
    - (e)   Picric acid type
    - (f)   Quinhydrone type

3. *Inclusion complexes*
    - (a)   Channel lattice type
    - (b)   Layer types
    - (c)   Clathrates
    - (d)   Monomolecular type

2.2   Metal Ion Complexes

A satisfactory understanding of metal ion complexation is based up on the familiarity with atomic structure and molecular forces. In this type metal ion constitutes the central atom (substrate) and interacts with a base (Electron pair donor, ligand). This type of interaction leads to the formulation of co-ordination bonds between the species.

2.2.1 Inorganic Complexes

This group constitutes the simple inorganic complexes first described by Werner in 1891. The ammonia molecules in hexamine cobalt III chloride, as the compound $[CO(NH_3)_6]^{3+}$ Cl_3^- is called ligands and are said to be coordinated to the cobalt ion. The coordination number of the cobalt ion (or) number of ammonia groups coordinated to the metal ion is six.

Other complex ions belonging to the inorganic group include $[Ag(NH_3)_2]^+$, $[Fe(CN)_6]^{4-}$ and $[Cr(H_2O)_6]^{3+}$.

Each ligand donates a pair of electrons to form a coordinate covalent link between itself and the central ion having an incomplete electron shell.

E.g.: $CO^{3+} + 6:NH_3 = [Co(NH_3)_6]^{3+}$

Werner has enumerated a number of rules by which some of the deviations from the classical theories of valency can be rationalised. According to Werner, postulates are given as follows:

1. There are two types of valencies

    (a) Primary (ionic)

    (b) Secondary (coordinate)

2. Same type of anion, radical or molecule may be held by either (or) both types of valences.

3. For each central atom or ion, there is a fixed number of Non-ionic valencies. The coordinated atoms or groups occupy the first sphere (or) coordinated sphere. Other atoms are said to be in the second (or) ionization sphere.

4. Neutral molecules as well as ions may satisfy non-ionic valences.

5. The non-ionic valences are directed towards definite positions in space (stereo isomerisation).

These postulates can be illustrated by the following example.

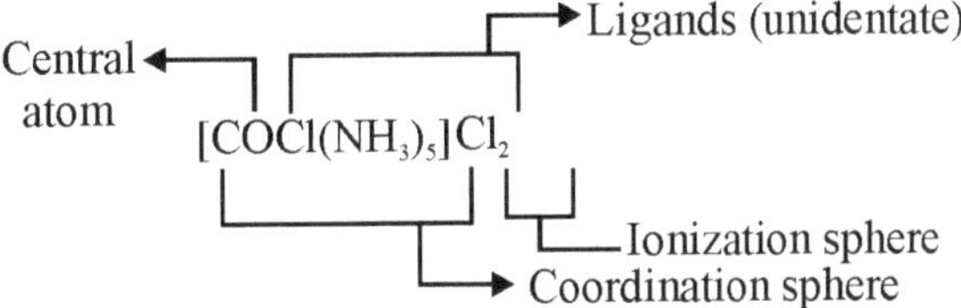

Explanation:

(a) In solution, this compound ionises to form $[CoCl(NH_3)_5]^{2+}$ and $2Cl^-$ ions.

(b) The chloride ion in the coordinated sphere cannot be precipitated by silver nitrate.

(c) Groups such as Cl, NH_3 in the coordinated sphere are called Ligands. They always donate electrons to the central atoms.

(d) The type of bonding between metal and ligand may be electrostatic (or) covalent.

The concept of hybridization can be extended to understand the formation of coordinated compounds of this type. Ligands donates a pair of electrons in forming a complex.

E.g.: H_2O: :NH_3 :NC   Cl:

This electron pair is accepted by metal ion. In metals, all the orbitals such as s, p, and d are to be considered to account the complexation.

The coordination number of cobalt is 6. The trivalent cobalt ion Co(III) has the given electronic configuration in the ground state.

Cobalt seems to make use of their 3d, 4s and 4p orbitals in forming hybrids, but this type is different from the classical concept of hybridization.

2.2.2 Chelates

A substance containing two or more donar groups may combine with a metal to a form a special type of complex known as chelate. Some of the bonds in a chelate may be ionic or covalent type, while others are coordinate type.

When the ligand provides one group for attachment to the central ion, the chelate is called as mono dentate. Pilocarpine behaves as mono dentate ligand toward Co(II), Ni(II) and Zn(II) to form chelates of Pseudo tetrahedral geometry.

Molecules with two or three donar groups are called bidentate and tridentate repetitively.

$$HOOC-H_2C \diagdown \quad \diagup CH_2-COOH$$
$$N-CH_2-CH_2-N$$
$$HOOC-CH_2 \diagup \quad \diagdown CH_2-COOH$$

EDTA

Ethylenediamine tetraacetic acid (EDTA) has six points of attachment to the metal ion and is known as hexadentate.

Vitamin B_{12} and hemo proteins are incapable of reacting with chelating agents, because their metal is already coordinated in such a way that only the trans position of the metal are available for complexation.

Chlorophyll and haemoglobin are the two compounds are naturally accruing chelates involved in the life processes of plants and animals.

In the process of sequestration, the chelating agent and metal ion to form a water-soluble compounds. EDTA is widely used to sequester and remove ca ions from hard water.

2.2.3 Olefin and Aromatic Type

These types of complexes are used as catalysts in the manufacture of bulk drugs, intermediates and in the analysis of drugs.

2.3   Organic Molecular Complexes

In this type of coordination complexes, components are organic molecules and these are held together by weaker forces or hydrogen bonding. The same components can also form molecular compounds when experimental conditions are altered.

In these complexes, the individual species are bound together by van der Walls force, dipole – induced dipole interactions and hydrogen bonding. The forces are weaker and the energy of attraction is less than 5 kcal/mole. The bond distance between the components is more than $30A^\circ$. Hence covalent bond is not involved.

Organic molecular complexes are classified as electron donar acceptor types and charge transfer complexes.

2.3.1 Donor-Acceptor Type

In this type, bond is between uncharged species, but lacks charge transfer. Dipole-dipole and London dispersion forces are responsible for its stability.

Example:

N-dimethylaniline and 2,4,6-trinitroanisole react in cold conditions to give a molecular complex.

These two compounds react at an elevated temperature to yield a salt, the constituent molecular of which are held together by primary valence bonds. The dotted line in the complex indicates that the two molecules are held together by a weak forces of interaction between the species.

2.3.2 Charge Transfer Complexes

In this type, one molecule polarizes the other. The resulting electrostatic interaction leads to the formation of the complex. Interactions between the species is ionic type. Resonance makes the main contribution for stability.

Electron drift or partial electron transfer by polarization

2.3.3 Drug and Caffeine Complexes

Higuchi and his associates have investigated the complexing of caffeine with a number of acidic drugs. The interaction between caffeine and a drug such as sulfonamides and barbiturates forms a complex due to dipole-dipole force or hydrogen bonding between the polarized carbonyl groups of caffeine and hydrogen atom of the acid. The interaction occurs between non-polar parts. This interaction leads to squeezing out the complex from the aqueous environment. Drugs such as benzocaine, procaine and tetracaine form complexes with caffeine. The mechanism of interaction is dipole-induced dipole type. The interaction is illustrated as follows.

Caffeine

Benzocaine

In the caffeine molecule, nitrogen at the 1 position can become more strongly electrophilic or acidic, owing to the withdrawal of electrons by the oxygen at position 2 and 6. The positive centre of nitrogen offers a site for complexation. In the benzocaine molecule, the ester become polarised in such a way that the carbonyl oxygen acts as a nucleophile. The complexation occurs as a result of induced dipole-dipole interaction between carboxy oxygen of benzocaine and electrophilic nitrogen of caffeine.

2.3.4 Polymer Complexes

Polyethylene glycols, polystyrene carboxy methyl cellulose and similar polymers containing nucleophilic oxygens can form complexes with various drugs. These can form complexes with various drugs such as carbowaxes, pluronics, tannic acid, salicylic acid and phenols.

This type of complexation produces incompatibilities in the dosage forms such as suspension, emulsions and ointments. Incompatibilities may delay the absorption, loss of preservative action and undesirable physical, chemical and pharmacological actions.

2.3.5 Picric Acid Complexes

Butesin picrate if used as a 1% ointment for burns and painful skin abrasions. In this complex, the antiseptic activity of picric acid is combined with the anesthetic activity of butesin.

Picric acid, being a strong acid, forms organic molecular complexes with weak bases, where as it combines with strong bases to yield salts such as 2 : 1 complex of butesin picrate is shown.

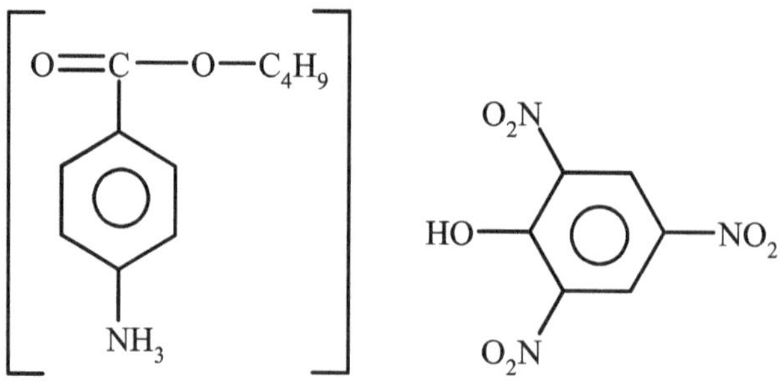

Picric acid is known to form complexes many carcinogenic agents.

2.3.6 Quinhydrone Complexes

The molecular complex of this type is obtained by mixing alcoholic solutions of equimolar quantities of benzoquinone and hydroquinone. The complex settles as green crystals. This complex can dissociate into individual components in an aqueous solution, when saturated. Therefore quinhydrone complex is used as an electrode in pH determination.

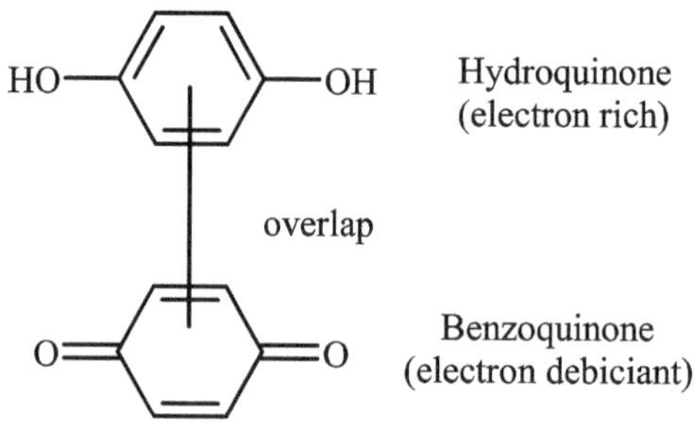

2.4   Inclusion Complexes

These complexes are also called as occlusion compounds in which one of the components is trapped in the open lattice or cage like crystal structure of the other. Here, the interaction is not due to chemical reactivity, but because of the favourable molecular architecture. The forces of are weaker.

2.4.1 Channel Lattice Type

The starch-iodine solution is a channel type of complex. In which the Iodine molecules are trapped within the spirals of the glucose molecules. The crystals of deoxycholic acid are arranged for forming a channel into which complexing molecule fits.

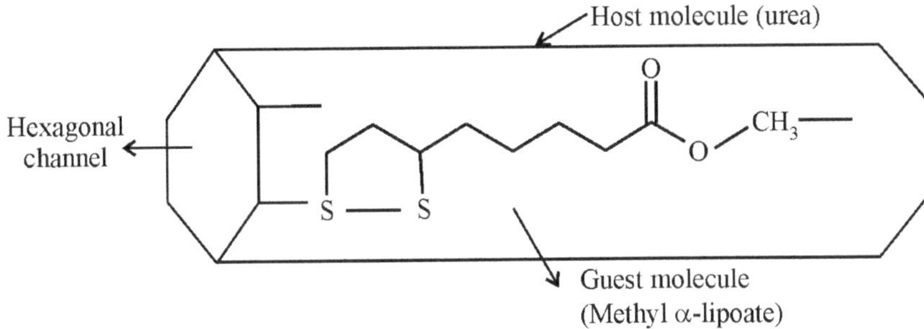

Fig. 2.1

Channel forming substances (host): Deoxycholic acid, urea, thiourea, amylase etc.

Guest agents: Paraffins, esters, acids, ethyl alcohol, dioxane etc.

Applications

1. Used for the separation of optical Isomers.

2. In the analysis of dermatological creams, long chain compounds may interfere with the assay methods.

2.4.2 Layer Types

Compounds such as clays, montmorillonite can entrap hydrocarbons, alcohols and glycols. They can form alternate monomolecular layers of guest and host.

2.4.3 Clathrates

Warfarin sodium USP is a clathrate of water and isopropyl alcohol. It is available as white crystalline powder. During crystallisation, certain substances form a cage like lattice in which the coordinating compound is entrapped.

Example

Hydroquinone molecules crystallize in the cage like structure with Hydrogen bonding.

The holes having a diameter of 4.2 $\overset{\circ}{A}$ and permit the entrapment of small molecules such as methyl alcohol, carbondioxide and hydrochloric acid.

Applications

1. Synthetic metal-alumino silicates are used as molecular sieves.

2. These materials are used to store gaseous volatile and toxic substances by the mechanism of clathrate.

2.4.4   Monomolecular Inclusion Complexes

Monomolecular inclusion compounds involve the entrapment of a single guest molecule in the cavity of one host molecule. Most of the host molecules are cyclodextrins. Cyclodextrins are cyclic oligosaccharides containing a minimum of six D-(+) gluco pyranase units, attached by 1,4 linkages.

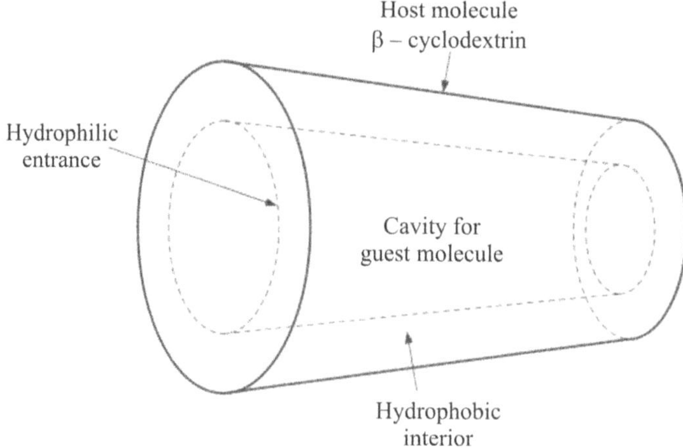

Fig. 2.2 Representation of cavity formed by β-cyclodextrin (Host molecule).

Applications

These types of complexes are studied for their uses in the design of dosage forms.

1. Enhanced solubility
2. Enhanced dissolution
3. Enhanced stability
4. Sustained release

2.5   Method of Analysis

The analysis of complexes involves the estimation of two parameters.

1. The stoichiometric ratio of ligand to metal or donar-to-acceptor.
2. Stability constant of the complex.

In order to achieve these objectives the following methods are used.

1. Method of Continuous Variation
2. Distribution Method
3. Solubility Method
4. pH Titration Method

1. Method of Continuous Variation: The physical properties such as dielectric constant, refractive index and spectrophotometric extinction coefficients are characteristics of particular species, when there is no complexation between these species (A and B), the value of property is additive. In case of complexation, these properties change, i.e., additive phenomena do not hold good changes in the dielectric constant on account of complexation.

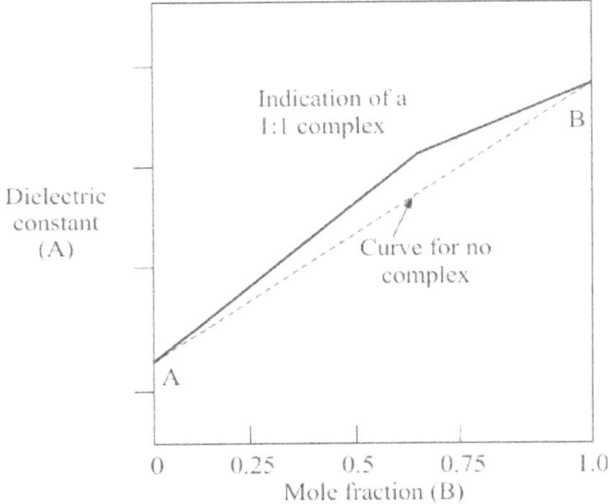

Fig. 2.3 Method of Continuous variation.

2. Distribution Method

The distribution of a solute between two immiscible liquids is expressed by distribution coefficient or partition coefficient. When a solute complexes with an added substance, the solute distribution pattern changes depending on the nature of a complex.

3. Solubility Method

When the components in a mixture produce a complex, the solubility of one of the components may be enhanced or inhibited. The change in solubility profile is taken as a criterion to decide the complexation behaviour. The experimental data can be used to analyse complexes in terms of donor-acceptor ratio and equilibrium stability constant. Based on the solubility profile, phase diagrams are classified as Type A and Type B. The examples for B solubility are:

Examples

D-Aminobenzoic acid (PABA) and caffeine, paracetamol and caffeine.

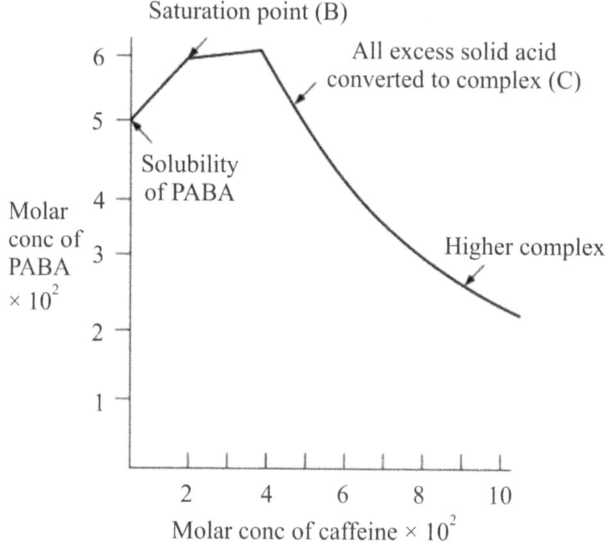

Fig. 2.4 The Solubility of para-amino benzoic acid in the presence of caffeine.

4. pH Titration Method

This method is used for the analysis of complexes provided such an interaction produces a change in the pH of the mixture.

Examples

Chelation of cupric ions by glycine molecules, chelation of calcium ions by EDTA.

Principle

The reaction can be represented by

$$Cu^{2+} + 2NH_3 + CH_2COO^- \rightarrow Cu(NH_2CH_2COO) + 2H^+$$

Since two protons are formed in the reaction complexation should result in the decrease in pH.

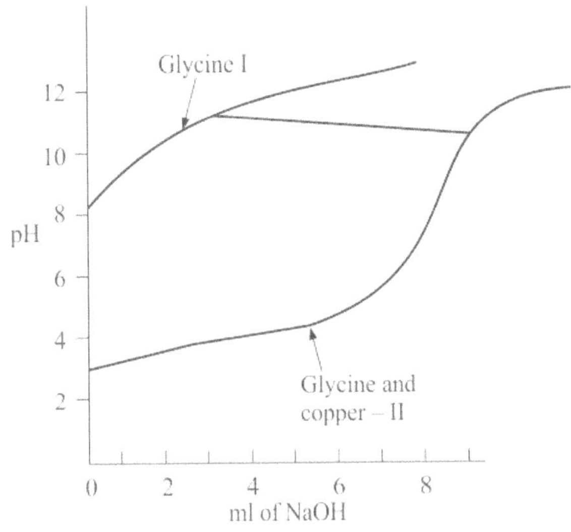

Fig. 2.5 Titration of glycine and glycine in the presence of cupric ions.

2.6   Applications of Complexation

Physical State: Liquid substance can be converted to solid substance to improve the processing characters with the help of complexation.

Example: Nitroglycerine can be converted into its crystalline complex with beta cyclodextrin. This complex contains 15.6% nitroglycerine and it is explosion proof.

Volatility: Complexation helps to overcome an unpleasant odour and it reduces substrate volatility by making complex.

Example: The formulation of povidone is form of a complex with polyvinyl pyrrolidone (PVP).

Solid State Stability: Sold state stability of drugs can be increased by complexation.

Example: Beta cyclodextrin complexes of vitamin A and D are stabilised chemically.

Vitamin A and D are stabilised chemically.

Chemical Stability: Complexation will change chemical reactivity, either by inhibitory (or) catalytic effect.

Example: The rate of hydrolysis of benzocaine can be reduced by complexing it with caffeine.

Solubility: There are many examples of solubility enhancement by complexation.

Example: At low concentrations, caffeine enhances the solubility of para-Amino Benzoic Acid (PABA).

Dissolution: Complexation is only the method by which both solubility and dissolution rate are increased (So, if solubility increases, the dissolution rate also increases).

Example: The dissolution rate of Phenobarbital is enhanced by using cyclodextrin inclusion complexes.

2.6.1 Partition Coefficients

Example: Permaganate ions in aqueous phase transferred into benzene phase by complexation with ether through ion-pair mechanism.

Absorption and Bioavailability: The absorption and bioavailability of tetracylines was reduced when administered with divalent cations like Ca^{+2}, Mg^{+2}, Al^{+3} by forming insoluble metal complexes.

Beta cyclodextrin complexes of indomethacin, barbiturates have the increased drug bioavailability.

Reduced Toxicity: Cyclodextrins are effective in reducing the ulcerogenic effect of indomethacin and local tissue toxicity of chlorpromazine.

Antidote for Metal Poisoning: Toxic metal ions like arsenic, mercury, antimony bind to –SH groups of various enzymes and interfere with their normal function.

Examples: Dimercaprol, form water soluble complex with these metal ions and eliminate them rapidly from the body. Other examples:

Beryllium poisoning -   Salicylic acid

Lead poisoning -   EDTA

Drug Action through Metal Poisoning: 8-hydroxy quinoline can form complex with iron i.e., present in the body, this complex can penetrate through the cell membrane of the malaria parasite leading to accumulation of excess metal in body and thus provide better anti-malarial action.

Anti-Bacterial Activity: Anti tubercular drug, PAS (Para Amino Salicylic Acid) forms a cupric complex, chelate cupric chelate has shown greater *in vivo* antitubercular activity in mice. Chelate is 30 times more fat soluble than the ionic complex, which is responsible for better penetration of drug into the cells of tubercle-bacilli.

Some complexes are available as drugs in the market. They are:

(a) *Cisplatin (DDP, Cis-Dichlorodiammine Platinum II, trade name – Platinol):* It is a co-ordination compound which has broad applications in human cancer chemotherapy. It has divalent platinum bound to chlorides. Two ammonia groups are irreversibly form a co-ordiante covalent bond, trans position to the chlorides.

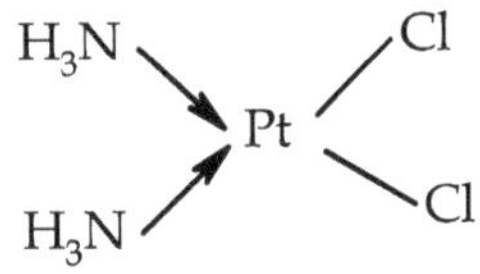

Cisplatin

(b) *Povidone – Iodine:* Polyvinyl pyrrolidone (PVP) is a water soluble polymer and forms a water soluble complex with iodine. As, the complex is soluble in water, drug can be removed easily from the site of application. Povidone Iodine is a safe and effective anti-bacterial and germicidal agent.

Uses: It is available as a soap for hand wash, surgical hand-scrub, skin preparations and also for wound cleansing, protection.

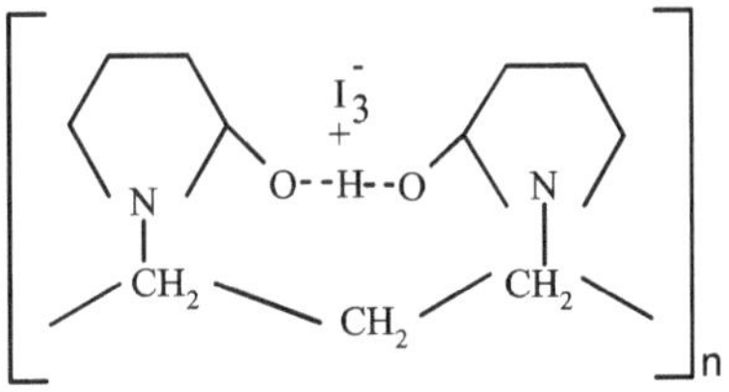

Povidone-Iodine Complex

Chapter 3

Chemical Kinetics

3.1 Chemical Kinetics

Chemical kinetics involves the study of the rate of a chemical process. The rate of a reaction can be understood by studying the time course of changes in the concentration.

The manufacturer is responsible for assuring the stability of marketed products, the community pharmacist also must have understanding of stability characteristics to handle and store products under proper conditions. He (or) she must also recognise that alterations may occur when a drug is combined with other ingredients.

Example

If thiamine hydrochloride, which is most stable at a pH of 2 to 3 and it is unstable above pH6 is combined with a buffered vehicle of pH 8 or 9 the vitamin is rapidly inactivated. Knowing the rate at which a drug deteriorates at various hydrogen ion concentration allows one to choose a vehicle that will retard or prevent the degradation.

3.1.1 Rates and Orders of Reactions

The rate, velocity or speed of a reaction is given by the expression, $\dfrac{dc}{dt}$, where dc is the increase or decrease of concentration over an infinitesimal time interval dt.

According to the law of mass of action, the rate of a chemical reaction is proportional to the product of the molar concentration of the reactants each raised to a power usually equal to the number of molecules a and b, of the substances A and B undergoing reaction.

In the reaction,

$$aA + bB + = \text{Products}$$

The rate of reaction is

$$\text{Rate} = \frac{-1}{a} \frac{d(A)}{dt}$$

$$= -\frac{1}{b}\frac{d(B)}{dt} = ...k(A)^a(B)^b....$$

$\therefore$ k = rate constant

The overall rate of a reaction is the sum of the exponents a + b of the concentration terms, A and B. The order with respect to one of the reactants, A or B, is the exponent a or b of that particular concentration term.

Example:

In the reaction of ethyl acetate with sodium hydroxide in aqueous solution.

$$CH_3COOC_2H_5 + NaOH \rightarrow CH_3COONa + C_2H_5OH$$

The rate expression is

$$R = -\frac{d[CH_3COOC_2H_5]}{dt}$$

$$= -\frac{d[NaOH]}{dt} = k[CH_3COOC_2H_5]^1[NaOH]^1$$

The reaction in first order (a = 1) with respect to ethyl acetate and first order (b = 1) with respect to sodium hydroxide solution, overall the reaction is second-order (a + b = 2).

In this case the contribution of sodium hydroxide to the rate expression is considered constant and the reaction rate can be written as

$$-\frac{d[CH_3COOC_2H_5]}{dt} = k^1[CH_3COOC_2H_5]$$

in which k^1 = K(NaOH). The reaction is said to be Pseudo-first order, it depends only on the first power (a = 1) of the concentration of ethyl acetate.

3.1.2   Molecularity

A reaction whose overall order is measured may be considered to occur through several steps or elementary reactions. Each of the elementary reactions has a stoichiometry giving the number of molecules taking part in that step. Since the order of an elementary reaction gives the number of molecules coming together to react in the step is known as molecularity of the elementary reactions.

Hence order and molecularity are identical only for elementary reactions. Bimolecular reactions may or may not be second order.

In simple terms, molecularity is the number of molecules, atoms or ions reacting in an elementary process. In the reaction.

$$Br_2 \rightarrow 2Br$$

The process is unimolecular, since the single molecule, Br_2, decomposes to form two bromine atoms. In the single step reaction

$$H_2 + I_2 \rightarrow 2HI$$

The process is bimolecular, since two molecules one of H_2 and one of I_2, must come together to form the product HI.

Termolecular reactions are proceeds in which three molecules must come together simultaneously. This is rare.

3.1.3 Specific Rate Constants

The constant (k) in the rate law associated with a single step reaction is called the specific rate constant for that reaction.

Example: Temperature, solvent (or) slight change in one of the reacting specific will lead to a rate law having a different value for the specific rate constant.

3.1.4 Units of Basic Rate Constant

The units for rate constants is expressed in terms of variables of the equation are

For zero order reactions

$$k = \frac{-dA}{dt} = \frac{moles\,/\,litre}{second}$$

$$= \frac{moles}{litre \times second} = moles\ litre^{-1}\ second^{-1}$$

For First-order reaction,

$$k = -\frac{dA}{dt}\frac{1}{A} = \frac{moles\,/\,liter}{second(moles\,/\,liter)}$$

$$= \frac{1}{second} = second^{-1}$$

For Second-order reaction,

$$k = -\frac{dA}{dt}\frac{1}{A^2} = \frac{moles\,/\,liter}{second(moles\,/\,liter)^2}$$

$$= \frac{liter}{mole \times second} = liter\ second^{-1} moles^{-1}$$

where A is the molar concentration of the reactant

3.2   Zero Order Reactions

Zero order reaction is defined as a reaction in which the rate does not depend on the concentration terms of the reactants.

This is mathematically expressed as

$$-dc\big/dt = k_o$$

where k_o is the specific rate constant for a zero order.

Examples

1.   Colour loss of liquid multi-sulfonamide preparation. Colour loss is proportional to decrease in the concentration.

2.   Oxidation of vitamin A in an oily solution.

3.   Photochemical degradation of chlorpromazine in aqueous solution.

In zero order reaction, the rate must depend on some factor other than the concentration term. The rate limiting factors are solubility in suspensions and absorption of light in photo chemical reactions.

The rate equation for zero order can be written as

$$\frac{-dA}{dt} = k_o \qquad\qquad .....(3.1)$$

In this reaction, the concentration is measured in terms of optical density. The negative sign indicates the colour fading. If eq. 3.1 is integrated, we get an equation that will permit the estimation of colour fading at any time (t).

Integrate eq. (3.1) between initial absorbance, A_0 at t = 0 time, and absorbance A_t at t = t.

$$\int_{A_0}^{A_t} dA = -k_0 \int_{0}^{t} dt$$

$$A_t - A_0 = -k_0 t$$

$$(\text{or})$$

$$k_0 = \frac{A_0 - A_t}{t} \qquad\qquad .....(3.2)$$

This is the Integral equation for zero order reaction. In general integral equation helps in estimating the reaction rate constant.

3.2.1 Half Life

It is time required for the concentration of the reactant to reduce to half of its initial concentration.

As per the definition, the equation can be written as

$$c = \frac{a}{2} \qquad t = t_{1/2}$$

The units of Half life period is sec/conc, min/conc, hr/conc etc.

3.2.2 Shelf Life

It is defined as the time required for the concentration of the reactant to reduce 90% of its initial concentration.

As per the definition the equation can be written as

$$C = \frac{90a}{100} \qquad t = t_{90}$$

3.2.3   Suspensions, Apparent Zero-Order Kinetics

Suspensions are another case of zero-order kinetics in which the concentration in solution depends on the drug solubility. As the drug decomposes in solution, more drug is released from the suspended particles, so that the concentration remains constant. This concentration is the drug equilibrium solubility in a particular solvent at a particular temperature.

The important point is that the amount of drug in solution remains constant despite its decomposition with time. The reservoir of solid drug in suspension is responsible for this constancy.

The equation for an ordinary solution, with no reservoir of drug to replace that depleted, the first order expression is

$$\frac{-d[A]}{dt} = k[A]$$

In which A is concentration of drug remaining undecomposed at time t and k is known as first order constant.

When the concentration (A) is constant, in case of suspension, we may write

$$K[A] = k_0$$

So that the first order rate law becomes

$$\frac{-d[A]}{dt} = k_0$$

This equation can be written as apparent zero-order kinetics

3.3   First Order Reaction

First order reaction is defined as a reaction in which the rate of reaction depends on the concentration of one reactant. This equation can be written as

$$\frac{-dc}{dt} = kc \qquad\qquad .....(3.3)$$

It shows that the decomposition rate of hydrogen peroxide is catalyzed by 0.02M KI was proportional to the concentration of the hydrogen peroxide remaining in the reaction mixture at any time. The data for the reaction is

$$2H_2O_2 \rightarrow 2H_2O + O_2$$

In the equation (3.3) in which c is the concentration of hydrogen peroxide remaining undecomposed at time t and k is the first order velocity constant.

Integrating above equation between concentration c_0 at time t = 0 and concentration (c) at some time (t) we have

$$\int_{c0}^{c} \frac{dc}{c} = k \int_{0}^{t} dt$$

$$ln\ c - ln\ c_0 = -k\ (t - 0)$$

$$ln\ c = ln\ c_0 - kt \qquad\qquad .....(3.4)$$

Converting to common logarithms yields

$$log\ c = log\ c_0 - kt/2.303 \qquad\qquad .....(3.5)$$

$$k = \frac{2.303}{t} log \frac{c_0}{c} \qquad\qquad .....(3.6)$$

In exponential form, the equation becomes

$$c = c_0\ e^{-kt} \qquad\qquad .....(3.7)$$

$$c = c_0^{\ 10^{-kt/2.303}} \qquad\qquad .....(3.8)$$

The concentration asymptotically approaches a final value c_∞ as time proceeds towards affinity

The equation can be written as

$$k = \frac{2.303}{t} log \frac{a}{(a-x)} \qquad\qquad .....(3.9)$$

In which the symbol a is customarily used to replace c_0, x is the decrease of concentration, in time (t) and $(a - x) = c$.

The linear expression in eq. (3.5) shows that the slope of the line is $-k/2.303$ from which the rate constant is obtained. If a straight line is obtained, it indicates that the reaction is first order as shown in the fig 3.1.

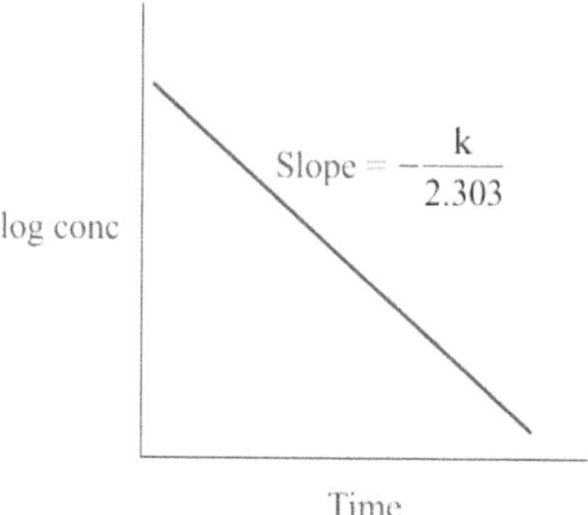

Fig. 3.1 Linear plot of log c *vs* time.

3.3.1 Half Life

The period of time required for a drug to decompose to one half the original concentration as calculated.

$$t_{1/2} = \frac{2.303}{k}\log\frac{500}{250} = \frac{2.303}{k}\log 2$$

$$t_{1/2} = \frac{0.693}{k}$$

3.4   Second Order Reactions

Second order reaction is defined as a reaction in which the rate depends on the concentration terms of two reactants each raised to the power on c.

$$A + B \rightarrow \text{Products}$$

Consider the rates of bimolecular reactions which occur when two molecules come together are frequently described by second order equation. When the speed of the reaction depends on the concentration of A and B with each term raised to the first power, the rate of decomposition of A, is equal to the rate of decomposition of B and both are proportional to the product of the concentration of the reactants.

$$\frac{-d[A]}{dt} = -\frac{d[B]}{dt} = k[A][B] \qquad .....(3.10)$$

If a and b are the initial concentrations of A and B and x is the concentration of each species reacting in time (t) the rate law may be written as

$$\frac{dx}{dt} = k(a-x)\,(b-x) \qquad .....(3.11)$$

in which dx/dt is the rate of reaction and (a – x) and (b – x) are the concentrations of A and B remaining at time (t); when in the simplest case both A and B are present in the same concentration so that a = b

$$\frac{dx}{dt} = k(a-x)^2 \qquad .....(3.12)$$

The eq.(3.12) is integrated by using the conditions that x = 0 at t = 0 and x = x at t = t.

$$\int_0^x \frac{dx}{(a-x)^2} = k\int_0^t dt$$

$$\left(\frac{1}{a-x}\right) - \frac{1}{(a-0)} = kt$$

$$\frac{x}{a(a-x)} = kt \qquad .....(3.13)$$

(or)

$$k = \frac{1}{at}\left[\frac{x}{a-x}\right] \qquad .....(3.14)$$

When in the general case, A and B are not present in equal concentrations, integration of eq. 3.13 yields.

$$\frac{2.303}{a-b}\log\frac{b(a-x)}{(b-x)} = kt$$

(or)

$$k = \frac{2.303}{t(a-b)}\log\frac{b(a-x)}{a(b-x)} \qquad .....(3.15)$$

where $\frac{x}{a}(a-x)$ is plotted against t, a straight line results if the reaction is second order. The slope of the line is k.

3.5   Determination of Order

The order of a reaction may be determined by several methods.

3.5.1 Substitution Method

The data accumulated in a kinetic study may be substituted in the integrated form   of the equations that describe the various orders when the equation is found in which the calculated k values remain constant within the limits of experimental variation.

3.5.2 Graphic Method

A plot of the data in the form of a graph shows a straight line results when concentration is plotted against t, the reaction is zero order. The reaction is first order if log (a – x) vs time yields a straight line and it is second order if $\frac{1}{(a-x)}$ vs t gives a straight line.

When a plot of $\frac{1}{(a-x)^2}$ against t produces a straight line, with all reactants at the same initial concentration, the reaction is third order.

3.5.3 Half-Life Method

In a zero-order reaction, the half-life is proportional to the initial concentration. The half life of a first-order reaction is independent of a; $t_{1/2}$ for a second-order reaction in which a = b is proportional to $\frac{1}{a}$ and in a third order reaction, in which a = b = c, it is proportional to $\frac{1}{a^2}$.

where

$$t_{1/2} \propto \frac{1}{a^{n-1}} \qquad \qquad .....(3.16)$$

in which n is the order of the reaction. Thus if two reactions are run at different initial concentrations, a_1 and a_2 the half-lives $t_{1/2}(1)$ and $t_{1/2}(2)$ are related as follows.

$$\frac{t_{1/2}(1)}{t_{1/2}(2)} = \frac{(d_2)^{n-1}}{(d_1)^{n-1}} = \left(\frac{d_2}{d_1}\right)^{n-1} \qquad \qquad .....(3.17)$$

Logarithmic form

$$\log \frac{t_{1/2}(1)}{t_{1/2}(2)} = (n-1)\log \frac{d_2}{dt} \qquad \qquad .....(3.18)$$

and finally

$$n = \frac{\log C t_{1/2}(1) / t_{1/2}(2)}{\log\left(\frac{d_2}{d_1}\right)} + 1 \qquad \qquad .....(3.19)$$

The half-lives are obtained graphically by plotting a *vs* t at two different initial concentrations and reading the time at $\frac{1}{2}a_1$ and $\frac{1}{2}a_2$.

3.6 Complex Reactions

Many reactions cannot be expressed by simple zero-first-second-third order equations. They involve more than one step (or) elementary reactions are known as complex reactions. These processes include revresible, parallel and consecutive reactions.

1. Reversible reaction

$$A + B \underset{k_{-1}}{\overset{k_1}{\rightleftharpoons}} C + D \quad \text{it is k and k–1}$$

2. Parallel (or) side reactions

$$A \begin{cases} \xrightarrow{\ K_1\ } B \\ \xrightarrow{\ K_2\ } C \end{cases}$$

3. Consecutive reactions

$$A \xrightarrow{\ k_1\ } B \xrightarrow{\ k_2\ } C$$

3.6.1 Reversible Reactions

The simplest reversible reactions is one in which both the forward and reverse steps are first-order processes.

$$A \underset{k_r}{\overset{k_f}{\rightleftharpoons}} B$$

According to this description, the net rate at which A decreases will be given by the rate at which A decreases in the forward step less the rate at which A increases in the reverse step.

$$\frac{-dA}{dt} = k_f A - K_r B \qquad \qquad .....(3.20)$$

The rate law may be integrated by noting that

$$A_0 - A = B \qquad \qquad .....(3.21)$$

Substitute the eq.(3.21) in eq.(3.20) affords, upon the integration,

$$ln\frac{k_f A_0}{\left(k_f + k_r\right)A - k_r A_0} = \left(k_f + k_r\right)t \qquad \qquad .....(3.22)$$

Eq.(3.22) may be simplified by introducing the equilibrium condition

$$K_f A_{eq} = k_r B_{eq} \qquad \qquad .....(3.23)$$

in which $\qquad \qquad A_0 - A_{eq} = B_{eq} \qquad \qquad .....(3.24)$

equation (3.23) and (3.24) may be used to solve for the equilibrium concentration in terms of the starting concentration

$$A_{eq} = \frac{k_r}{k_f + k_r} A_0 \qquad \qquad .....(3.25)$$

$$ln\frac{A_0 - A_{eq}}{A - A_{eq}} = \left(k_f - k_r\right)t \qquad \qquad .....(3.26)$$

(or)

$$log\frac{A_0 - A_{eq}}{A - A_{eq}} = \frac{\left(k_f + k_r\right)}{2.303}t \qquad \qquad .....(3.27)$$

The equation (3.27) has the advantage that the approach of A to equilibrium can be followed over a much wider range of concentrations than if an attempt is made to obtain the first order rate constant k_f in the early stages of the reaction when $B \approx 0$. The equation corresponds to a straight line intersecting at zero and having a slope given by $\frac{k_f + k_r}{2.303}$. Since the equilibrium constant of the reaction is given by

$$k = \frac{k_f}{k_r} - \frac{B_{eq}}{A_{eq}}$$

Both the forward and reverse rate constants can be evaluated once the slope of the line and the equilibrium constant are have been determined.

3.6.2 Parallel or Side Reactions

Parallel reactions are common in drug systems, particularly when organic compounds are involved.

The base catalyzed degradation of prednisolone will be used to illustrate the parallel type process.

Gutmann and Meister investigated the degradation of the steroid prednisolone in aqueous solutions containing sodium hydroxide as a catalyst.

This was carried at 35 °C.

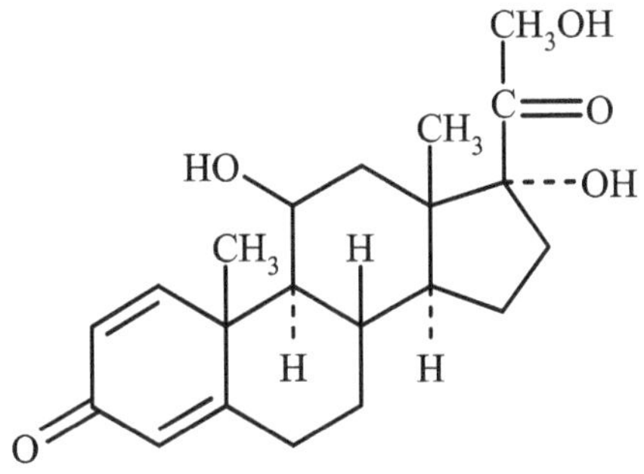

Prednisolone

In which $k = k_1 + k_2$, the first order equation is integrated to give

$$ln\left(P_0/P\right) = kt \qquad\qquad .....(3.28)$$

$$P = P_0 e^{-kt} \qquad\qquad .....(3.29)$$

The rate of formation of the acidic product can be expressed as

$$\frac{dA}{dt} = k_1 P = k_1 P_0^{e-kt} \qquad\qquad .....(3.30)$$

Integrating of equation yields

$$A = A_0 + \frac{k_1}{k} P_0 \left(1 - e^{-kt}\right) \qquad\qquad .....(3.31)$$

In which A is the conc. of the acid product at t and A_0 and P_0 are the initial conc. of the acid and prednisolone respectively.

$$A = \frac{k_1}{k} P_0 \left(1 - e^{-kt}\right) \qquad\qquad .....(3.32)$$

For the neutral product,

$$N = \frac{k_2}{k} P_0 \left(1 - e^{-kt}\right) \qquad\qquad .....(3.33)$$

The equation 3.32 and 3.33 shows a suggest that for the base-catalyzed break down of prednisolone, a plot of the conc. A (or) N against $(1 - e^{-kt})$ should yield a straight line.

3.6.3 Series or Consecutive Reactions

These reactions are common in radioactive series in which a parent isotope in decay by a first order process in to daughter isotope.

The depletion of glucose in acid solution may be represented as

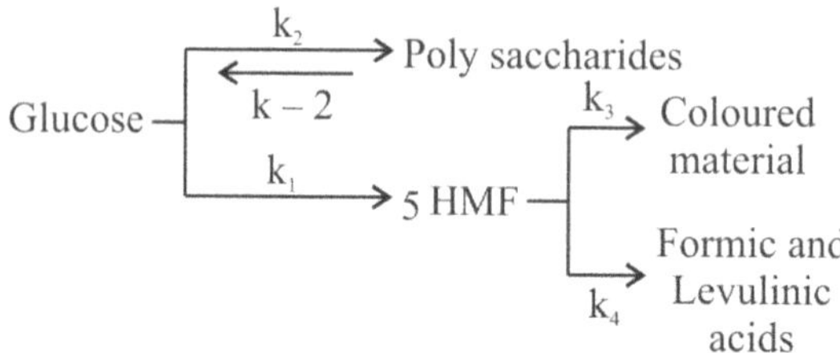

which is such in all types of complex type reactions – reversible, parallel and consecutive process.

$$A \xrightarrow{k_1} B \xrightarrow{k_2} C$$

in which A is Glucose, B is 5-HMF and C is final break down product. The rate of decomposition of glucose is given by

$$-dA/dt = k_1 A \qquad \qquad .....(3.34)$$

The rate of change in concentration of 5-HMF is

$$dB/dt = k_1 A - k_2 B \qquad \qquad .....(3.35)$$

Break down product is

$$dc/dt = k_2 B \qquad \qquad .....(3.36)$$

Integration take place

$$A = A_0 e^{-k_1 t} \qquad \qquad .....(3.37)$$

$$B = \frac{A_0 k_1}{k_2 - k_1}\left(e^{-k_1 t} - e^{-k_2 t}\right) \qquad \qquad .....(3.38)$$

The rate constants k_1 and k_2 and concentrations of break down products (c) can be determined.

3.7   The Steady State Approximation

3.7.1 Michaelis – Menten Equation

The steady state approximation is commonly used to reduce the labour in deducing the form of a rate flow. We will illustrate this approximation by deriving the Michaelis-Menten equation.

Michaelis and Menten assumed that the interaction of a substrate S with an enzyme E to yield a product (P) followed by reaction sequence given by

$$E + S \underset{k_2}{\overset{k_1}{\rightleftharpoons}} (E-S) \xrightarrow{k_3} P$$

According to this the rate of product formation

$$\frac{dP}{dt} = k_3 (E.S) \qquad \qquad .....(3.39)$$

The rate of formation of (E.S) is $\dfrac{d(E.S)}{dt} = k_1(E)(S) - k_2(E.S) - k_2(E.S) \qquad .....(3.40)$

(or)

$$\frac{d(E.S)}{dt} = k_1(E)(S) - (k_2 + k_3(E.S) \qquad \qquad ......(3.41)$$

If the concentration of E.S is constant throughout most of the reaction and is always much less than the concentration of S and P, we can write

$$\frac{d(E.S)}{dt} = 0 \qquad \qquad .....(3.42)$$

It follows from equation (3.41) and (3.42) that

$$(E.\ S)_{ss} = \frac{k_1(E)(S)}{k_2 + k_3} \qquad \qquad .....(3.43)$$

In which the subscript (E. S) is used to designate the concentration referred as steady-state value.

The total concentration of enzyme E_0 is the sum of the concentration of enzyme, both free E and bound E.S

$$E = E + (E.\ S) \qquad\qquad .....(3.44)$$

Eliminating E from eq. (3.42), (3.43) and (3.44) we obtain

$$\left(E.S\right)_{ss} = \frac{k_1 S E_o}{\left(k_2 + k_3\right) + k_1 S} \qquad\qquad .....(3.45)$$

(or)

$$\left(E.S\right)_{ss} = \frac{S E_o}{k_m + S} \qquad\qquad .....(3.46)$$

In which $\qquad\qquad k_m = \dfrac{k_2 + k_3}{k_1} \qquad\qquad .....(3.47)$

Thus, under steady-state conditions, the rate of product formation is given by

$$\frac{dP}{dt} = \frac{k_3 S E_0}{k_m + s} \qquad\qquad .....(3.48)$$

which may be recognized as Michaclis-Menten equation

From eq. (3.39) dp/dt becomes v_m and $v_m = k_3\ E_0$, since E.S is equivalent to E_0 according from eq.(3.48)

$$v = v_m \frac{S}{k_m + S} \qquad\qquad .....(3.49)$$

From eq.(3.49) may be used to obtain a linear expression, known as Lineweaver-Burk equation.

$$\frac{1}{v} = \frac{k_m + S}{v_m . S}$$

$$\frac{1}{v} = \frac{1}{v_m} + \frac{k_m}{v_m}\frac{1}{S} \qquad\qquad .....(3.50)$$

From eq. (3.50), we see that a plot of $\dfrac{1}{v}\ vs\ \dfrac{1}{S}$ yields a straight line with an intercept on the vertical axis of $\dfrac{1}{v_m}$ and a slope of $\dfrac{k_m}{v_m}$.

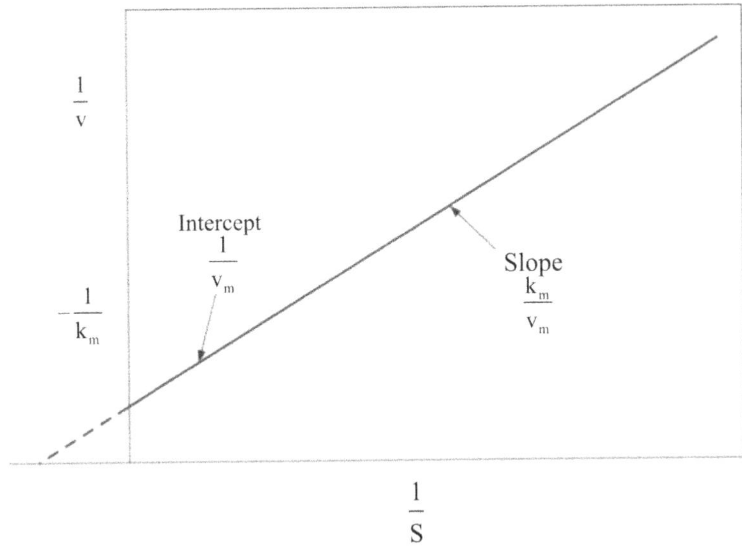

Fig. 3.2 A Lineweaver-Burk plot of Michaelis-Menten kinetics showing the calculation of k_m by two means.

3.8   Influence of Temperature and other Factors on Reaction Rates

3.8.1   Temperature

A number of factors other than concentration may affect the reaction velocity. Among these temperature, solvents, catalysts and light. The speed of many reactions increases about two to three times with each 10 °C rise in temperature. The effect of temperature on reaction rate is given by the equation.

$$k = A_e - {E_a}/{RT} \qquad\qquad .....(3.51)$$

(or)

$$\log k = \log A - \frac{E_a}{2.303} - \frac{1}{RT} \qquad\qquad .....(3.52)$$

In which k is the specific reaction rate, A is a constant known as the Arrhenius factor or frequency factor, E_a is the energy activation, R is the gas constant 1.987 calories/deg mole, and T is the absolute temperature.

3.8.2   Classic Collision Theory of Reaction Rates

The Arrhenius equation is an empiric relation giving the effect of temperature on an observed rate constant. Relations of this type are observed for unimolecular and bimolecular reactions and also observed for complex reactions involving a number of bimolecular and unimolecular steps. The temperature dependence of complex reactions, and uni and bimolecular reactions appear to reflect a physical requirement that must be met for a reaction occur.

The manner by which temperature affects molecular motion may be understood by considering a hypothetic situation in which all the molecules of a substance are moving in the same direction at the same velocity.

If a molecule deviates from its course it will collide with another molecule, causing both molecules to move off in different directions with different velocities. A chain of collision between molecules can occur, which finally results in random motion of all the molecules.

The kinetic energy is proportional to the square of velocity, the distribution of molecular velocities corresponds to the distribution of molecular energies, and the fraction of the molecules having a given kinetic energy can be expressed by the Boltzmann distribution law.

$$f_i = \frac{N_i}{N_T} = e^{-E_i/RT} \qquad .....(3.53)$$

From the Boltzmann distribution law, we note that of the total number of moles N_T of a reactant, N_i moles have a kinetic energy given by E_i.

The rate of a reaction can be considered proportional to the number of moles of reactant having sufficient energy to react, that is

$$\text{Rate} = PZN_i \qquad .....(3.54)$$

(P) the probability constant gives that a collision between molecules will lead to the product.

Substituting for N_i in eq. (3.54) yields

$$\text{Rate} = (PZ)\, e^{-E_iRT}\, N_T \qquad .....(3.55)$$

which, when compared with the general rate law

$$\text{Rate} = k$$

$$k = (PZ)e^{-E_iRT} \qquad ......(3.56)$$

Thus, collision state theory interprets the Arrhenius factor A in terms of the frequency of collision between molecules and

$$A = PZ \qquad .....(3.57)$$

The Arrhenius activation energy E_a as the minimum kinetic energy a molecule must possess in order to undergo reaction

$$E_a = E_i$$

3.8.3 Transition State Theory

Transition state theory is also absolute rate theory, according to which an equilibrium is considered to exist between the normal reactant molecules and an activated complex of these molecules.

Decomposition of the activated complex of these molecules leads to product. For an elementary bimolecular process, the reaction may be written as

$$A + B \Rightarrow [A.......B]^{+} \rightarrow P$$

Normal reactant   Activated reactant   Product molecules
molecules

3.8.4 Effect of the Solvent

The influence of solvent on the rate of decomposition of drugs is a topic of great importance to the pharmacist. The reaction of non-electrolytes related to the internal pressure or solubility parameters of the solvent and solute.

The influence of ionic strength and dielectric constant of the medium on the rate of ionic reactions are also significant.

3.8.5 Influence of Dielectric Constant

The effect of the dielectric constant on the rate constant of an ionic reaction, extrapolated to infinite dilution, where the ionic strength effect is zero. It is also useful for the preparations of new drugs.

$$ln\, k = ln\; k_{\epsilon} = \infty \;\; -\frac{NZA^{2}Be^{2}}{RTr}\; \frac{1}{\epsilon}$$

where

$k_{\epsilon} = \infty$ is the rate const in a medium of infinite dielectric constant

N = Avogadro's number

Z_A and Z_B = charges on the two ions

e = dielectric constant

r = Distance between ions in the activated complex

ϵ = Dielectric constant of the medium

3.8.6 Catalysis

The rate of reaction is frequently influenced by the presence of catalyst. The hydrolysis of sucrose in the presence of water at room temperature proceeds with a decrease in the energy. When the H_2 ion concentration is increased by adding small amount of acid, inversion proceeds at a measurable rate.

A catalyst is defined as a substance that influences the speed of a reaction without being altered chemically. When a catalyst decreases the velocity of a reaction it is called a negative catalyst.

Since catalyst remain unaltered at the end of a reaction, it does not change the overall ΔG° of the reaction hence, according to the relationship

$$\Delta G^\circ = - RT \, ln \, k$$

The catalyst combines with the reactant known as substrate and forms an intermediate known as complex.

Specific Acid-Base Catalysis

Solutions of a number of drugs undergo accelerated decomposition up on the addition of acids or bases. If the drug solution is buffered, the decomposition may not be accompanied by an appreciable change in the concentration of acid or base. So that the reaction is may be considered to be catalyzed by hydrogen or hydrogen ions. When the rate law for such an accelerated decomposition is bound to contain a term involving the concentration of hydrogen ion or concentration of hydroxyl ion, the reaction is said to be specific acid-base catalysis.

General Acid-Base Catalysis

In this process, buffers are used to maintain the solution at a particular pH. In addition to the effect of pH on the reaction rate, there may be catalysis by one or more species of the buffer components. The reaction is said to be general acid or general base catalysis.

Whether the catalytic components are acidic or basic, the pH profile of a reaction that is susceptible to general acid base catalysis.

3.9   Pseudo First Order Reaction

Pseudo first order reaction which is originally a second order, but is made to behave like a first order reaction.

In second order reaction, the rate depends on the concentration terms of two reactants. Therefore the rate equation would be

$$\frac{-dc}{dt} = k_2 \left[A\right]\left[B\right] \qquad .....(3.58)$$

where A and B are the reactants in the reaction and k_2 is the second order constant. Therefore, the concentration of (B) does not change significantly during the course of the reaction then the eq. (3.58) changes to

$$\frac{-dc}{dt} = k_2[A][\text{cons}\tan t] = k_1[A]$$

Thus the rate depends on the concentration of one reactant (on a), i.e., first order reaction. This type of reaction is also termed as apparent first order.

Examples

Hydrolysis of ester is catalyzed by H^+ ions. Here the concentration of H^+ ions remains constant. Therefore, the rate solely depends on the concentration of the ester.

- Base-catalyzed oxidative degradation of prednisolone in aqueous solution.
- Acid catalyzed hydrolysis of erythromycin oxime.
- Acid catalyzed hydrolysis of digoxin.

3.10   Decomposition and Stabilization of Medicinal Agents

Pharmaceutical decomposition can be classified as hydrolysis, oxidation, isomerization, epimerization and photolysis and these processes may effects the stability of drugs in liquid, solid and semisolid products. This may effects the ingredients of dosage forms and environmental factors may have an effect on chemical and physical stability of pharmaceutical preparations.

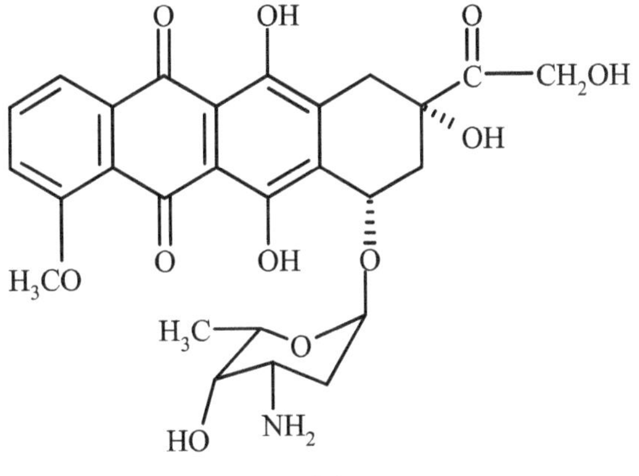

Doxorubicin

Beijnen investigated the stability of doxorubicin in aqueous solution using a stability indicating high performance liquid chromatography (HPLC) assay procedure. Doxorubicin has been used as various human neoplasms for the past 20 years.

The degradation of mitomycin c in acid solution was studied by Beijnen and Underberg. Mitomycin c shows both strong antibacterial and antitumor activity. Degradation in alkaline solution involves removal of an amino group and replacement by a hydroxyl group, but the breakdown of mitomycin c is more complicated in acid solutions, involving ring opening and the formation of two isomers, namely trans and cis mitosene.

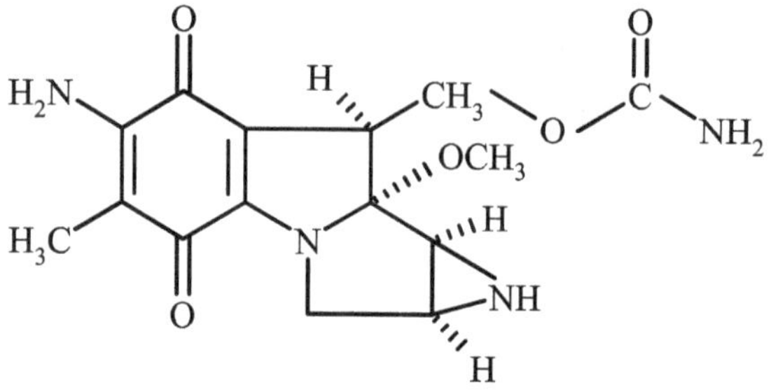

Mitomycin C

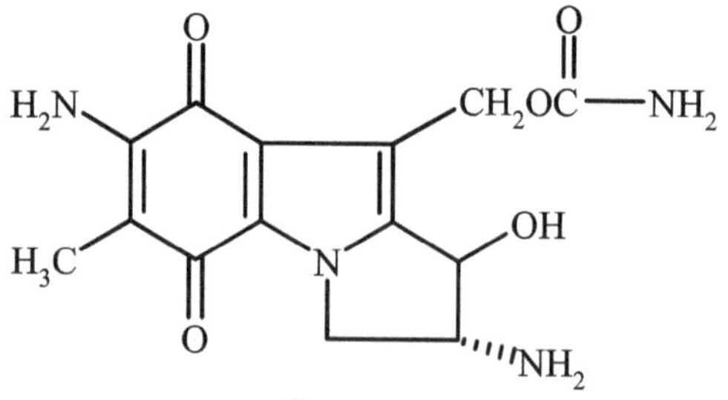

I

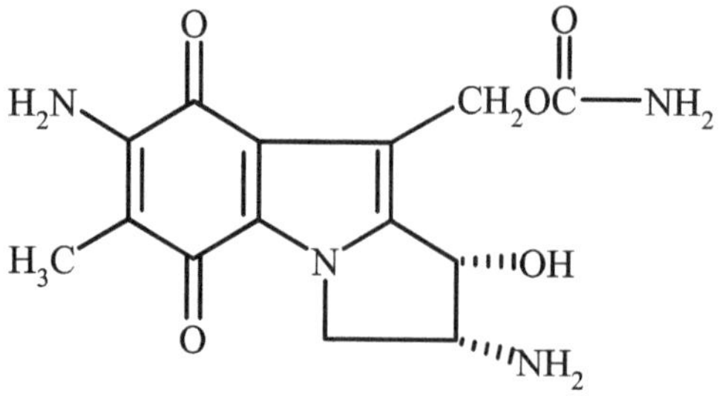

II

To study the mechanism of degradation the authors designed an HPLC assay that allows quantitative separation of the parent drug and its decomposition products. The kinetics of mitomycin c in acid solution was studied at 20 °C. To obtain pH values below 3 the solutions were acidified with aqueous perchloric acid are having pH 3-6 they were buffered with acetic acid acetate buffer. The degradation of mitomycin c shows first order kinetics over a period of more than 3 half lives.

3.10.1   Influence of Light in Photodegradation

Light is not classified as catalyst and its effect on chemical reactions is treated as a separate topic. Light energy like heat, may provide the activation necessary for a reaction to occur. Radiation of the proper frequency and energy must be absorbed to activate the molecules. The energy unit of radiation is known as the photon and is equivalent to 1 quantum of energy. Photochemical reactions do not depend up on the temperature for activation of the molecules. So, the rate of activation is independent of temperature.

The study of photochemical reactions requires strict attention to control the wavelength and intensity of light and number of photons actually absorbed by the material. Reactions that occur by photochemical activation are usually complex and proceed by a series of steps.

Examples of photochemical reactions of interest in pharmacy and biology are the irradiation of ergosterol and the process of photosynthesis when ergosterol is irradiated with light in the ultraviolet region, vitamin D is produced. In photosynthesis, carbon dioxide and water are combined in the process of a photosensitizer, chlorophyll absorbs visible light and light then brings about the photo chemical reaction in which carbohydrates and oxygen are formed.

The second class of photooxidation is initiated by a dye such as methylene blue.

The photooxidation of benzaldehyde in n-decane solution showed that the reaction involved a free radical mechanism. More proposed to show whether a free radical process occurred in dilute aqueous solution and to study the antioxidant efficiency of polyhydric phenols. The photooxidation of benzaldehyde was bound to follows catechol > Pyrogallol > hydroquinone > resorcinol > n-propyl gallate. These antioxidants could be classified as retarders rather than inhibitors for they showed the rate of oxidation, but did not inhibit the reaction.

The scheme of initiation, propagation and termination of the chain reactions are as shown.

$$\text{PhCHO} + h\nu \longrightarrow \text{Ph}\overset{\bullet}{\text{C}}\text{O} + \text{H}^{\bullet}$$

Initiation

$$\text{Ph}\overset{\bullet}{\text{C}}\text{O} + O_2 \xrightarrow{k_2} \text{Ph}\overset{\bullet}{\text{C}}\text{O}_3$$

Propagation

$$\text{Ph}\overset{\bullet}{\text{C}}\text{O}_3 + \text{PhCHO} \xrightarrow{k_3} \text{PhCO}_3\text{H} + \text{Ph}\overset{\bullet}{\text{C}}\text{O}$$

Propagation

$$2\ \text{Ph}\overset{\bullet}{\text{C}}\text{O}_3 \xrightarrow{k_4} \text{inert products}$$

Termination

Steps in Photooxidation of Benzaldehyde

3.11   Accelerated Stability Studies

Accelerated studies at high temperatures were used by most companies, but the criteria were often arbitrary and were not based on fundamental kinetic principles. For example, some companies used the rule that the storage of liquids 37 °C accelerated the decomposition at twice the normal temperature rate, while other manufacturers assume that it accelerated the breakdown by 20 times normal (Levy) has pointed out that such arbitrary temperature coefficients of stability cannot be assigned to all liquid preparations and other classes of pharmaceuticals.

The method of accelerated testing of pharmaceutical products based on the principles of chemical kinetics. According to this technique the (k) values for the decomposition of a drug in solution at various elevated temperatures are obtained by plotting conc. against time.

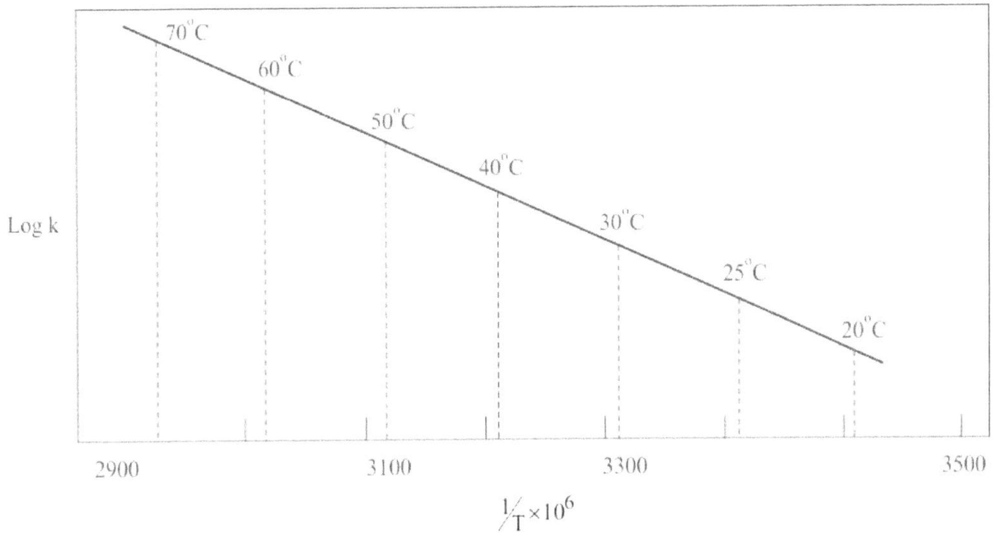

Fig. 3.3 Arrhenius plot for predicting drug stability of room temperature.

$$t = \frac{2.303}{2.09 \times 10^{-5}} \log \frac{94}{45} = 3.5 \times 10^4 \, hr \cong 4 \, yeatrs$$

Free and Blythe and more recently, and his associates have suggested a similar method in which the fractional life-period is plotted against the reciprocal temperatures and time in days required for the drug to decompose to fraction of its original potency at room temperature is obtained.

The log percent of drug remaining is plotted against time in days, and the time for the potency to fall to 90% of the original value (i.e., t_{90}) is read from the graph (Fig 3.4 and 3.5).

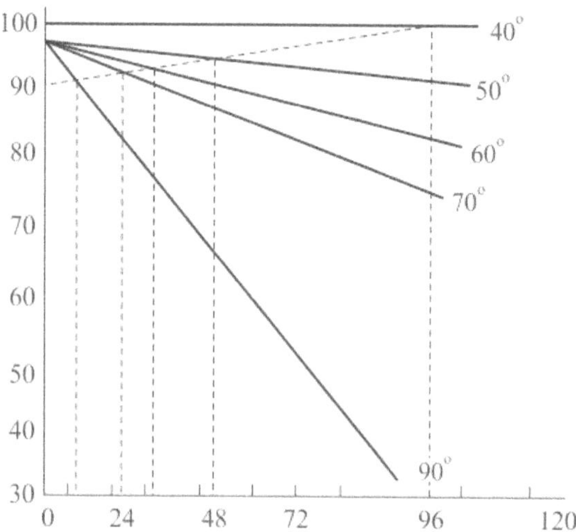

Fig. 3.4 Time in days required for drug potency to fall to 90% of original value.

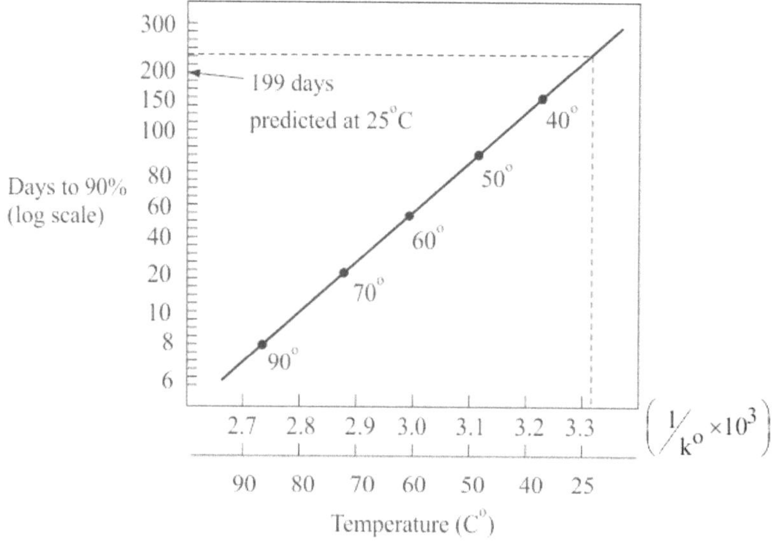

Fig. 3.5 A log plot of t_{90} against reciprocal of temperature.

The log time to 90% is then plotted against $\dfrac{1}{T}$ and the time at 25 °C gives the shelf life of the product in days.

An improved approach for stability evaluation is non isothermal kinetics, introduced by Rogers in 1963. The activation energy, reaction rates and stability predictions are obtained by programming the temperature to change at a predetermined rate. The temperature and time are related through an appropriate function.

Such as

$$\frac{1}{T} = \frac{1}{T_0} + at \qquad \qquad .....(3.59)$$

T_0 = Initial temperature

a= reciprocal heating rate constant

At any time during the run, the Arrhenius equation for time zero and time t may be written

$$ln\ kt = ln\ k_0 - \frac{E_a}{R}\left(\frac{1}{T_t} - \frac{1}{T_0}\right) \qquad \qquad .....(3.60)$$

By substituting eq. (3.59) and (3.60) yields

$$ln\ kt = ln\ k_0 - \frac{E_a}{R}(dt) \qquad \qquad .....(3.61)$$

Since temperature is a function of the time (t) a measure of stability k_t is directly obtained over a range of temperatures.

CHAPTER 4

INTERFACIAL PHENOMENA

4.1 Adsorption at Solid Interfaces

If a solid comes into contact with a gas or a liquid there is an accumulation of gas or liquid molecules at the interface i.e., the densities of the gas or liquid at the interface are greater than their bulk densities. This phenomenon is known as adsorption.

4.1.1 Adsorption

It involves penetration of the absorbing material by the molecules of the absorbed substance.

Adsorption on solid surface is of 2 types

1. Solid-vapour (Gas)
2. Solid-liquid (Adsorption)

General Applications of Adsorption

1. In the removal of gas, objectionable odours from rooms and food.
2. In the operation of gas masks.
3. In the measurement of the dimensions of particles in a powder.
4. In decolorizing solutions, in adsorption chromatography, detergency and wetting.

Types of absorption depends on nature of forces involved

1. Physical adsorption – Van der Waals forces
2. Chemisorptions – chemical bonds.

4.1.2 Solid-Gas Interface

The degree of adsorption of a gas by a solid depends on the chemical nature of the adsorbent (the material used to adsorb the gas) and adsorbate (the substance being adsorbed), the surface area of the adsorbent, the temperature, the partial pressure of the adsorbed gas.

Physical adsorption associated with vander Waals force is reversible the removal of the adsorbate from the adsorbent being known as desorption.

A physically adsorbed gas can be desorbed from a solid by increasing the temperature and reducing the pressure.

Chemisorptions in which the adsorbate is attached to the adsorbent by primary chemical bonds are be reversible unless the bonds are broken.

The relationship between the amount of gas physically absorbed on a solid and the equilibrium pressure or concentration at constant temperature yields an adsorption isotherm.

The term isotherm refers to a plot at constant temperature.

The characteristics of physical adsorption and chemisorption

S. No.	Property	Physical	Chemisorption
1.	Adsorption	Weak physical forces (Van der Waals forces) Heat of adsorption is usually < 50 kJ/mole. May be regarded as a surface condensation.	Involves transfer or sharing of electrons between adsorbent and adsorbed molecules. Heat of adsorption is usually about 60-420 KJ/mole may be regarded as surface tension.
2.	Specificity	Non-specific i.e., will occur to some degree in any system.	Specific i.e., only occurs when reaction is possible between adsorbent and adsorbate.
3.	Reversibility	Reversible i.e., adsorbate can be removed easily from surface is an unchanged form.	Often irreversible i.e., adsorbate is removed with difficulty usually is a changed form. E.g.: oxygen adsorbed by carbon is removed as carbondioxide.
4.	Effect of Temperature	Process is exothermic i.e., amount of adsorption decreases with rise in temperature	Surface reaction only proceeds above a certain temperature. Reaction is usually exothermic.
5.	Number of adsorbed Layers	Monomolecular layer formed at low pressures followed by additional layers as pressure increases. Condensation of vapour in capillaries of porous solid may occur.	Restricted to formation of a monolayer
6.	Rate of adsorption	Usually rapid at all temperatures	Usually proceed at a finite rate which increases rapidly with rise in temperature.

The number of moles, grams or millilitres 'x' of gas adsorbed on 'm' grams of adsorbent at STP is plotted on the vertical axis against the equilibrium pressure of the gas in mmHg on the horizontal axis as seen in Fig. 4.1(a).

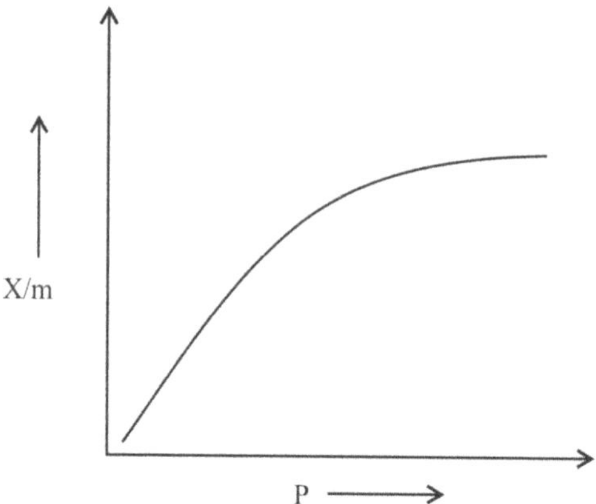

Fig. 4.1(a) Adsorption isotherm (Type I).

One method of obtaining adsorption data is by the use of an apparatus which consists essentially of a balance contained within a vacuum system. The solid, previously degassed is placed on the pan and known amounts of gas arc allowed to enter. The increase in weight at the corresponding equilibrium gas pressures is recorded. This can be achieved by noting the extension of a calibrated quartz spring used to suspend the pan containing the sample. The data are then used to construct an isotherm based on one or more of the following equations.

Freundlich suggested a relationship, the Freundlich isotherm.

$$y = \frac{x}{m} = kp^{1/n} \qquad \qquad ....(4.1)$$

where   y = mass of gas

x = adsorbed per unit mass

m = mass of adsorbent

k, n = constants that can be evaluated from the results of the experiment

The equation is handled more conveniently when written in logarithmic form,

$$\log \frac{x}{m} = \log k + \frac{1}{n} \log p \qquad \qquad ....(4.2)$$

which yields a straight line when plotted as seen in Fig. 4.1(b).

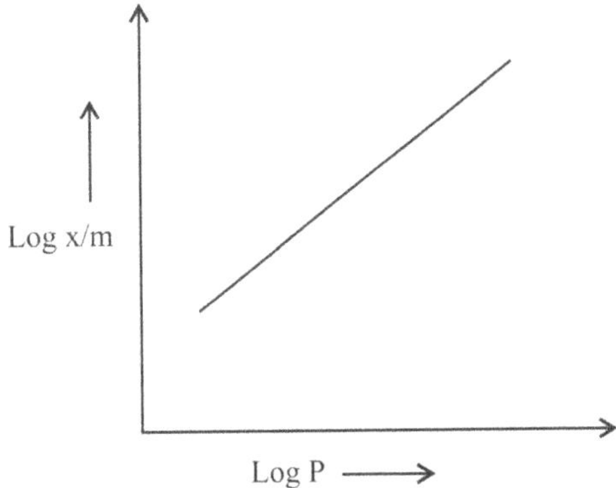

Fig. 4.1(b) Adsorption isotherm.

The constant,   log k, = Intercept on the ordinate

$1/n$ = slope of the line

Langmuir developed an equation based on the theory that the molecules or atoms of gas are adsorbed on active sites of the solid to form a layer one molecule thick (monolayer). The fraction of centres occupied by gas molecules at pressure p is represented by θ.

Fraction of sites not occupies = $1 - \theta$

The rate r_1 of the adsorption or condensation of gas molecules on the surface is proportional to the unoccupied spots, $1 - \theta$ and to the pressure, p on

$$r_1 = k_1 (1 - \theta)\, p \qquad \qquad ....(4.3)$$

The rate r_2 of evaporation of molecules bound on the surface is proportional to the fraction of surface occupied 'θ' ; or

$$r_2 = k_2 \theta$$

and at equilibrium, $r_1 = r_2$

or

$$k_1 (1 - \theta)p = k_2 \theta$$

by rearrangement we get

$$\theta = \frac{k_1 p}{k_2 + k_1 p} = \frac{(k_1 / k_2)\, p}{1 + (k_1 / k_2)\, p} \qquad \qquad ....(4.4)$$

we can replace k_1/k_2 by b

θ by y/y_m

where

y = mass of gas adsorbed per gram of adsorbent at pressure p and at constant temperature.

y_m = mass of gas that log of the adsorbent can adsorb when monolayer is complete.

Inserting these terms into equation (4.4), we get

$$y = \frac{y_m\, b_p}{1 + b_p} \qquad \qquad ....(4.5)$$

which is known as Langmuir isotherm. By inverting equation (4.5) and multiplying through by p, we can write this for plotting as

$$\frac{p}{y} = \frac{1}{b y_m} + \frac{p}{y_m} \qquad \qquad (4.6)$$

A plot of p/y against p should yield a straight line and y_m and b can be obtained from the slope and intercept.

Equations (4.1), (4.2), (4.5), (4.6) are adequate for the description of curves only of the type shown in Fig. (4.1a). This is known as Type-I isotherm.

Extensive experimentation has shown that there are four other types of isotherms as shown in Fig. (4.1c-f).

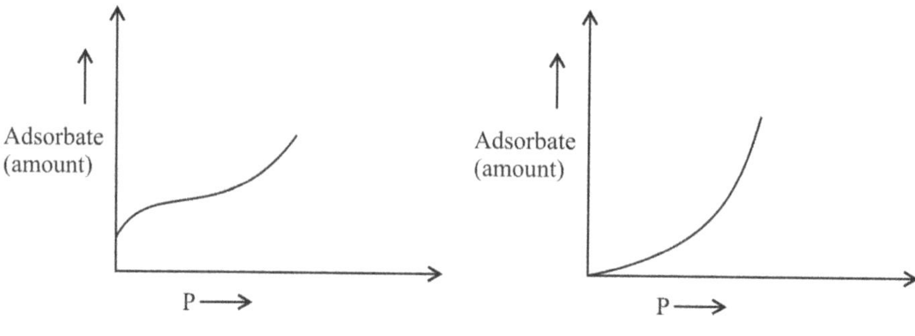

Type II Adsorption Isotherm   Type III Adsorption Isotherm

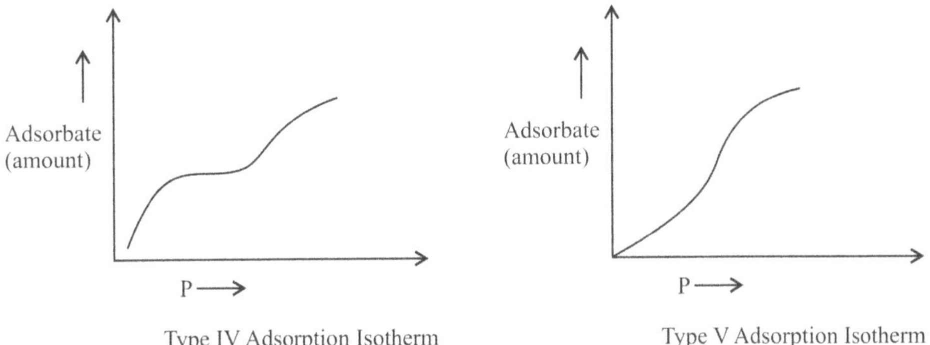

Fig. 4.1 (c - f) Type- II - V Adsorption isotherms.

Type-II

Type-II isotherms are sigmoidal is shape and occur when gases undergo physical adsorption onto nonporous solids to form monolayer followed by multilayer formation. The first inflection point represents formation of mono layer.

Type-II isotherms are best described by BET equation.

$$\frac{p}{y\,(p_0 - p)} = \frac{1}{y_m b} + \frac{(b-1)}{y_m b}\,\frac{p}{p_0} \tag{4.7}$$

where $p =$ pressure of the adsorbate in mmHg.

$m =$ mass of 'y' vapour per gram of adsorbent is adsorbed.

$p_0 =$ vapour pressure when the adsorbent is saturated with adsorbate vapour

$y_m =$ quantity of vapour adsorbed per unit mass of adsorbent when the surface is covered with a monomolecular layer.

$b =$ constant proportional to the different between the heat of adsorption of the gas in the first layer and the latent heat of condensation of successive layers.

Type-III, Type-V

Type-III, Type-V isotherms are produced in a relatively few instances in which the heat of adsorption of the gas in the first layer is less than the heat of condensation of successive layers.

Type-IV isotherms are observed on porous solids

Type-II isotherm results when $b > 2.0$

Type-III when $b < 2$ is BET equation

Types IV and V frequently involve hysteresis and appear as Fig. (4.1e), (4.1f).

4.1.3 Applications of Isotherms

1. The total surface area of solid can be determined from those isotherms in which formation of a monolayer can be detected, that is types I, II and IV.

2. This information is obtained by multiplying the total number of molecules in the volume of gas adsorbed by cross sectional area of each molecule.

4.1.4 The Solid-Liquid Interface

Drugs such as dyes, alkaloids, fatty acids and even inorganic acids and bases can be adsorbed from solution onto solids such as charcoal and alumina.

The adsorption of strychnine, atropine, quinine from aqueous solutions by six different clays was capable of being expressed by the Longmuir equation in the form

$$\frac{c}{y} = \frac{1}{by_m} + \frac{c}{y_m} \qquad (4.8)$$

where

c = equilibrium concentration in milligrams of alkaloidal base per 100 ml of solution

y = amount of alkaloidal base ($y = x/m$)

x = in milligrams adsorbed per gram, m of clay

b, y_m = constants

Barr and Arnista investigated the adsorption of diphtheria toxin and several bacteria by various clays. They concluded that attapulgite a hydrous magnesium aluminium silicate was superior to kaolin as an intestinal adsorbent. The results of the adsorption of strychnine on activated attapulgite, halloysite and kaolin all washed with gastric juice are shown in Fig. (4.1g).

The smaller the slope, better is the adsorption.

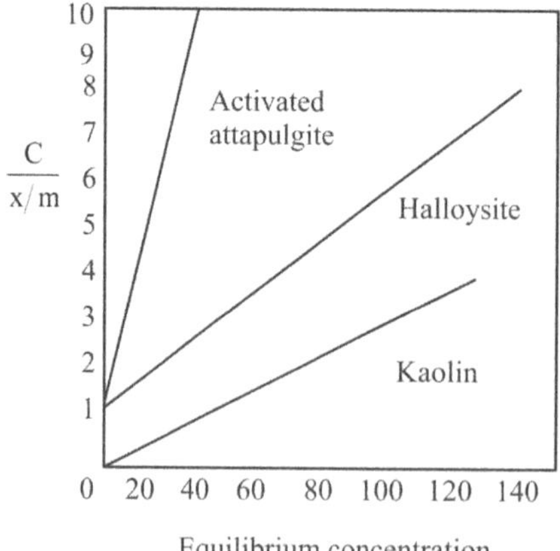

Fig. 4.1 (g) Adsorption isotherm representing adsorption at solid liquid interface.

4.1.5 Electric Properties of Interfaces

It deals with surfaces that are charged in relation to their surrounding liquid environment.

Particles dispersed in liquid media may become charged mainly in one of two ways.

1. It involves the selective adsorption of a particular ionic species present in solution. This may be an ion added to the solution or in case of pure water it may be the hydronium or hydroxyl ion. The majority of particles dispersed in water acquire a negative charge due to preferential adsorption of hydroxyl ion.

2. Charges on particles arise from ionization of groups (such as COOH) that may be situated at the surface of the particle. In these cases, the charge is a function of pK and pH.

3. Less common origin for the charge on a particle surface is thought to arise when there is a difference in dielectric constant between the particle and its dispersion medium.

4.1.6 The Electric Double Layer

Consider a solid surface in contact with a polar solution containing ions, for example, an aqueous solution of an electrolyte. Further more, let us suppose that some of the cations are adsorbed onto the surface giving it a positive charge. Remaining in solution are the rest of the cations plus the total number of anions added. These anions are attracted to the positively charged surface by electric forces that also serve to repel the approach of any further cations once the initial adsorption is complete. In addition to these electric forces, thermal motion tends to produce an equal distribution of all the ions in solution. As a result, an equilibrium situation is setup in which some of the excess anions approach the surface, whereas the remainder are distributed in decreasing amounts as one proceeds away from the charged surface. At a particular distance from the surface, the concentration of anions and cations are equal that is conditions of electric neutrality prevail. It is important to remember that the system as a whole is electrically neutral, even though there are regions of unequal distribution of anions and cations.

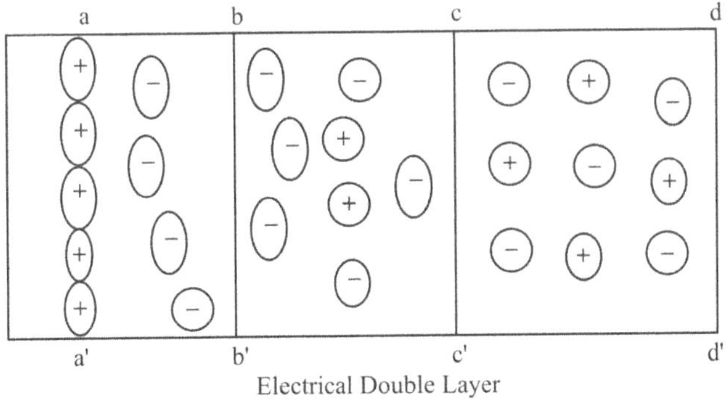

Fig. 4.1(h) Electrical double layer.

Such a situation is shown in where

$$aa^1 \Rightarrow \text{surface of solid}$$

The adsorbed ions that give the surface its positive charge are referred to as the potential-determining ions. Immediately adjacent to this surface layer is a region of tightly bound solvent molecules, together with some '–ve' ions also tightly bound to the surface. The limit of this region is given by the line bb^1. These ions having a charge opposite to that of potential-determining ions are known as counter ions or gengen ions. The degree of attraction of the surface is moved relative to the liquid, the shear plane is bb^1 rather than aa^1, the true surface.

In the region bounded by the lines bb^1 and cc^1, there is an excess of negative ions. The potential at bb^1 is still positive because as previously mentioned there are fewer anions in the tightly bound layer than cations adsorbed onto the surface of the solid. Beyond cc^1, the distribution of ions is uniform and electric neutrality is obtained. Thus, the electric distribution at the interface is equivalent to a double layer of charge, the first layer (extending from aa^1 to bb^1) tightly bound and a second layer (from bb^1 to cc^1) that is more diffuse. The so called diffuse double layer therefore extends from aa^1 to cc^1.

Two situations other than that represented in Fig. (4.1h) are possible.

(a)   If the counter ions in the tightly bound solvated layer equal the positive charge on the solid surface, then electric neutrality occurs at the plane bb^1 rather than cc^1.

(b)   Should the total charge of the counter ions is the region aa^1-bb^1 exceed the charge due to the potential-determining ions, then the net charge at bb^1 will be negative rather than less positive as shown in Fig (4.1h). This means that in this instance for electric neutrality to be obtained at cc^1, an excess of positive ions must be present in the region bb^1-cc^1.

4.1.7   Nernst and Zeta Potentials

The changes in potential with distance from the surface for the various situations can be represented as shown in Fig. (4.1h). The potential at the solid surface aa^1, due to potential determining ion is the electrothermodynamic (Nernst) potential and is defined as the difference in potential between the actual surface and the electro neutral region of the solution. The potential located at the shear plane bb^1 is known as the electro kinetic or zeta potential ζ. The zeta potential is defined as the difference in potential between the surface of the tightly bound layer and electro neutral region of the solution. As shown in Fig. (4.1h), the potential initially drops off rapidly followed by a more gradual decrease as the distance from the surface increases. This is because the counter ions close to the surface act as a screen that reduces the electro static attraction between the charged surface and those counter ions further a way from the surface. The zeta potential has practical application in the stability of systems containing dispersed particles because this potential, rather than the Nernst potentials governs the degree of repulsion between adjacent similarly charged dispersed particles. If the zeta potential is reduced below a certain value (which depends on the particular system being used) the attractive forces exceed the repulsive force and the particles come together. This phenomenon is known as flocculation.

4.1.8 Wetting Agent

A wetting agent is a surfactant which when dissolved in water, lowers the contact angle, aids in displacing an air phase at the surface and replaces it with a liquid phase.

In this case the behaviour of the liquid will depend on the balance between the forces of attraction between the solid and liquid phases and forces of attraction in the liquid molecules.

E.g.: 1. Mercury and glass

> In this example the forces of attraction between the mercury and glass are lesser than the forces of attraction between the mercury molecules themselves

2. Water and glass

> In contrast to the above example the attractive forces between solid and liquid molecules are greater than forces between molecules of liquid themselves.

> The most important action of a wetting agent is to lower the contact angle between the surface and wetting liquid.

4.1.9 Contact Angle

The angle between a liquid droplet and the surface over which it spreads.

Complete wetting may be signified by a contact angle $0°$ or $180°$ between a liquid and a solid.

Young's Equation

$$\gamma_s = \gamma_{SL} + \gamma_L \cos \theta \qquad \qquad \text{.....(4.9)}$$

$$s = \gamma_L (\cos \theta - 1) \qquad \qquad \text{.....(4.10)}$$

Alternative form of young's equation

$$w_a = w_{SL} = \gamma_L (1 + \cos \theta) \qquad \qquad \text{.....(4.11)}$$

where s = spreading coefficient

γ_s = interfacial tension at solid surface

γ_{SL} = interfacial tension at solid-liquid interface

θ = contact angle

To exhibit a low contact angle, the wetting agent should have an HLB of about 6-9.

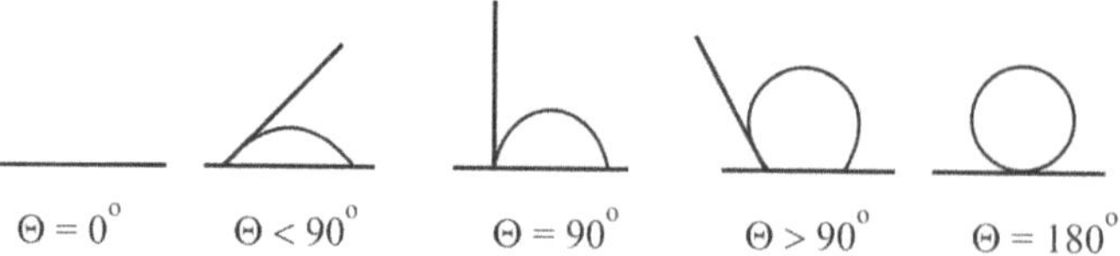

Fig. 4.1(i) Contact angles.

Zisman's Concept for Contact Angle

According to his experimental studies, the cosine of the contact angle, cos θ plotted versus the surface tension for a homologous series of liquids spreads on a surface such as Teflon, a straight line was observed. The line can be extraplotted to cos θ = 1 i.e., to a contact angle of zero, signifying complete wetting.

Critical surface Tension

The surface tension at cos θ = 1 was given the term critical surface tension and symbol γ_c.

Zisman concluded that γ_c was characteristic for each solid.

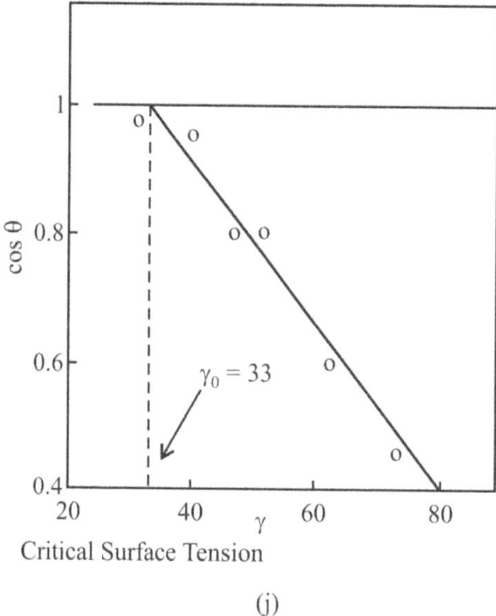

Fig. 4.1(j) Representation of critical surface tension.

E.g.: Teflon $\rightarrow \gamma_c = 18$ ergs/cm^2

Teflon is having $- CF_2 -$ groups.

Zisman reasoned that all surfaces of this nature ($-CF_2-$ groups) have critical surface tensions of about 18 ergs/cm^2.

Wetting Agent ability to enhance Spreading Coefficient

Draves Test involves the measuring of time for a weighted skin of cotton yarn to sink through the wetting solution contained in a 500 ml graduate.

Detergents

Detergents are surfactants that are used for the removal of dirt.

Detergency is a complex process involving the removal of foreign matter from surfaces

The detergency is a complex process which include:

- Initial wetting of the dirt and of the surface to be cleaned
- Deflocculation and suspension
- Emulsification or solubilization of the dirt particles
- Foaming of the agent for entrainment and washing away of the particles of dirt.

A detergent should posses a combination of all these properties.

4.1.10 Applications of Surfactants

- Emulsifying agents, detergents, wetting agents and solubilizing agents.
- Used as antibacterial and protective agents and as aids for the absorption of drugs in the body.
- A surfactant may affect the activity of a drug or may itself exert drug action.

  E.g.: penetration of the hexyl resorcinol into the pinworm, Ascaris is increased by the presence of a low concentration of the surfactant. This potentiation of activity is due to a reduction in interfacial tension between the liquid phase and the cell wall of the organism.

  When the concentration of surfactant exceeds than that required to form micelles rate of penetration of anthelmentic activitydecreases nearly to zero.

  E.g.: Quarternary ammonium compounds, they themselves possess antibacterial activity.

  These agents are absorbed on the cell surface and bring about destruction of the cell by increasing the permeability or leakiness of lipid cell membrane. Death of cell then occurs due to loss of essential materials from the cell.

Cationic Quaternary Ammonium Compounds

Both gram positive and gram negative organisms are susceptible to the action of these compounds.

Anionic Quaternary Ammonium Compounds

These agents attack gram positive organisms more easily than the gram negative bacteria.

Non ionic Surfactants

These are least effective as antibacterials.

4.1.11   Rat-gat Perfusion Technique

Miyamotol *et al.,* studied the effects of surfactants and bile slats and their effect on gastro intestinal absorption of antibiotics using this technique. Polyoxyethylenelauryl ether reduced the absorption of propilcillin in the stomach and increased it in the small intestine.

Some surfactants increases the rate of intestinal absorption where as some decrease it.

Applications of Wetting to Pharmacy and Medicine

- Displacement of air from the surface of sulphur, charcoal and other powders for the purpose of dispersing these drugs in liquid vehicles.
- Displacement of air from the matrix of cotton pads and bandages so that medicinal solutions can be absorbed for the application to various body areas.
- Displacement of dirt and debris by the use of detergents in the washing of wounds and application of medicinal lotions and sprays to the surface of the skin and mucous membrane.

CHAPTER 5

COLLOIDS AND MACROMOLECULAR SYSTEMS

5.1 Introduction

A disperse phase system consists essentially of one component. The disperse phase is dispersed as particles or droplets throughout another components the continuous phase.

The word colloid was coined by Graham in 1861 from the Greek word "Rodla" (means glue).

5.1.1 Definition

"The dispersions in which the size of the dispersed particles is within the range of 10^{-9} m (1 nm) to about 10^{-6} m (1 μm) are termed as colloids".

However the upper size limit is often extended to include emulsions and suspensions which are very polydispersed systems in which the droplet size frequently exceeds 1 μm, but which show many of the properties of colloidal systems. Many natural systems such as suspensions of microorganisms, blood and isolated cells in culture are also colloidal dispersions.

Some examples of colloidal systems of pharmaceutical interest are given in Table 5.1. Based on the size of the dispersed phase, three types of dispersed systems are generally considered. (a) molecular dispersions (b) colloidal dispersions and (c) coarse dispersions. The size range of these classes and their associated characteristics are given in Table 5.2. Colloidal dispersions are more stable usually than coarse dispersions since the larger particles in the latter settle rapidly under the influence of gravity and unlike colloidal systems, the maintenance of their dispersions is not aided by Brownian movement.

Table 5.1 Types of colloidal systems

Dispersion medium	Dispersed phase	Colloid type	Examples
Solid	Solid	Solid sol	Pearls, opals
Solid	Liquid	Solid emulsion	Cheese, butter
Solid	Gas	Solid foam	Pumice, marshmallow
Liquid	Solid	Sol. Gel	Jelly, paint
Liquid	Liquid	Emulsion	Milk, mayonnaise
Liquid	Gas	Foam	Shaving cream
Gas	Solid	Solid aerosols	Smoke, dust
Gas	Liquid	Liquid aerosols	Clouds, mist, fog

Table 5.2 Classification of dispersed systems based on particle size

Class	Range of particle size	Characteristics of System	Examples
Molecular dispersion	Less than 1 nm	Invisible in electron microscope. Pass through ultrafilter and semipermeable membrane rapid diffusion	Oxygen molecules, ordinary ions, glucose
Colloidal dispersion	From 1 nm to 0.5 μm	Visible in electron microscope, pass through filter paper but not semipermeable membrane. Diffuse very slowly	Colloidal silver solutions, neutral and synthetic polymer, cheese, butter, jelly, milk etc.
Coarse dispersion	Greater than 0.5 μm	Visible under microscope. Do not pass through filter paper and through semipermeable membrane. Do not diffuse	Grains of sand, RBC, most pharmaceutical emulsions and suspensions

5.2 Classification of Colloids

On the basis of interaction between the particles or macromolecules of the dispersed phase with the molecules of the dispersion medium, colloidal systems are classified into three groups.

1. Lyophilic – solvent "loving" colloidal in which the disperse phase is dissolved in the continuous phase,
2. Lyophobic – solvent "hating" colloids in which the disperse phase is insoluble in the continuous phase, and
3. Association colloids in which the dispersed phase molecules are soluble in the continuous phase and spontaneously "self assemble" or "associate" to form aggregates in the colloidal size range.

5.2.1 Lyophilic Colloids

Dissolution of acacia of gelatin in water or celluloid in amyl acetate leads to the formation of a solution. This is an example of this class as the disperse phase is dissolved in the continuous phase. The attachment of solvent molecules to molecules of the dispersed phase is due to attraction between the dispersed phase and the dispersion medium. This is termed as "Hydration" in case of hydrophilic colloids in which water is the dispersion medium. Most lyophilic colloids are organic molecules, for example gelatine, acacia, insulin, albumin, rubber and polystyrene of these first four produce lyophilic colloids in aqueous dispersion media (hydrophilic solution). Rubber and polystyrene forms lyophilic colloids in non-aqueous, organic solvents. These materials are referred to as lipophilic colloids. A material that forms lyophilic colloidal system is one liquid (e.g.: water) may not do so in another liquid (benzene).

5.2.2 Lyophobic Colloids

They differ from lyophilic colloids due to the absence of a solvent sheaths around the particle. Lyophobic colloids are generally composed of inorganic particles dispersed in water. Examples of such materials are gold, silver, sulphur, arsenous sulphide and silver iodide.

The preparative methods for lyophobic colloids may be divided into those methods that involve the breakdown of larger particles into particles of colloidal dimensions (dispersion methods) and these in which the colloidal particles are formed by aggregation of smaller particles such as molecules (condensation methods).

5.3   Dispersion Methods

The breakdown of coarse material may be affected by several means.

Colloid mills: These mills cause the dispersion of coarse materials by shearing in a narrow gap between a static cone and a rapidly rotating cone.

Electrical dispersion (bredig's method): Certain materials may be dispersed by the passage of an electric are between electrodes made of the metal and immersed in the dispersion medium.

Ultrasonic irradiation: The passage of ultrasonic waves through a dispersion medium produces alternating regions of cavitations and compression in the medium. The cavities collages with great force and cause the breakdown of coarse particles dispersed in the liquid.

Peptisation: Because the charges necessary for stabilising colloidal dispersions may originate from the preferential adsorption of specific ions at the surface of the particles, a finely divided solid may be converted into a colloidal dispersion by the addition of such ions to the dispersion medium. This process is known as peptisation.

Condensation methods: These involve the rapid production of supersaturated solutions of the colloidal material under conditions in which it is deposited in the dispersion medium as colloidal particles and not as precipitate. The supersaturation is often obtained by means of a chemical reaction that results in the formation of the colloidal material. For example, colloidal silver iodide may be obtained by reacting together dilute solutions of silver nitrate and potassium iodide; colloidal sulfur is produced from sodium thiosulfate and hydrochloric acid solutions; and ferric chloride boiled with excess of water produces colloidal hydrated ferric oxide.

A change of solvent may also cause the production of colloidal particles by condensation methods. If a saturated solution of sulfur in acetone is poured slowly into hot water, the acetone vaporizes, leaving a colloidal dispersion of sulfur. A similar dispersion may be obtained when a solution of a resin such as benzoin in alcohol is poured into water.

5.4   Purification of Colloids

5.4.1 Dialysis

Colloidal particles are too large to diffuse through the pores of certain membranes such as cellophane. The smaller particles in true solution are able to pass through these membranes. Dialysis method is used to separate micro molecular impurities from colloidal dispersions. The process is known as dialysis.

A colloidal dispersion may become diluted during dialysis because water pass through the membrane under the influence of the osmotic pressure of the colloid. Such dilution may be prevented by applying to the colloid a pressure that is equal to or greater than its osmotic pressure. This procedure is referred to as dialysis under pressure.

5.4.2 Electro Dialysis

An electrical potential may be used to increase the rate of movement of ionic impurities through a dialysing membrane and so provide a more rapid means of purification. This method is of little use if any of the impurities are uncharged and care should be taken to ensure that the electrical potential does not effect the stability of the colloid.

5.4.3   Ultrafiltration

Colloidal particles are too small to be retained by ordinary filter papers. In filtration through dialysing membrane the rate of flow of the liquid dispersion medium is slow so it is carried out under the influence of positive pressure or vacuum. Since the sizes of the colloidal particles and the pores in the membrane are so small the process is referred to as ultrafiltration.

It is possible to manufacture membrane with different droppers of porosity. The use of a series of ultrafilters with gradually decreasing pore size allows the particle size of a colloid to be determined. The pore size of an ultrafilter can be determined by the use of a series of colloidal dispersions of different particle sizes.

5.4.3 Association Colloids

The third type of colloids is association or amphiphilic colloids. Association colloids are aggregates or "associations" of amphipathic surface active molecules. These molecules are soluble in the solvent and their molecular dimensions are below the colloidal size range. When present in solution at concentration above a certain critical value (the CMC), these molecules tend to form association colloids. These aggregate which may contain 50 or more monomers are called micelles. The concentration of monomers at which micelles formed is termed the critical micelle concentration (CMC). The number of monomers that aggregate to form a micelle is known as the aggregation number of the micelle.

The phenomenon of micelle formation can be explained as follows. Below the CMC, the concentration of amphiphiles undergoing adsorption at the air-water interface increases as the air-water increases as the total concentration of amphiphiles is raised. Eventually a point is reached at which both the interface and the bulk phase become saturated with monomers. This is the CMC. Any further amphiphiles added in excess of this concentration aggregates to form micelles in the bulk phase and in this manner the free energy of the system is reduced.

In the case of amphiphiles in water, the hydrocarbon chains face inward into the micelle to form, hydrocarbon core. Surrounding this core are the polar portions of the amphiphiles associated with the water molecules of the continuous phase. Aggregation also occurs in non polar liquids. The orientation of the molecules is now reversed. These situations are shown in Fig. 5.1.

Amiphiphiles may be anionic, cationic, non ionic or ampholytic (Twitter ionic) and this provides a means of classifying association colloids. A typical example of each type is given in Table 3. Thus Fig. 5.1represents the micelle of an anionic association colloid. A certain number of the sodium ions are attracted to the surface of the micelle reducing the overall negative charge somewhat. These bound ions are called gegenious.

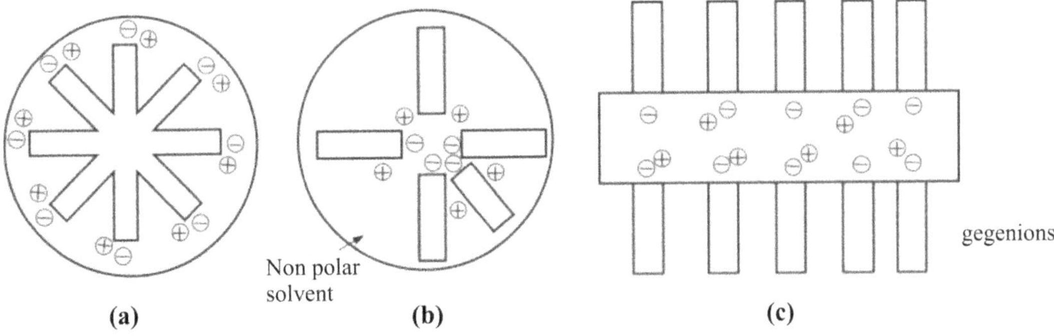

Fig. 5.1 Some probable shapes of micelles

(a) Spherical micelle in aqueous media,
(b) Reversed micelle in non-aqueous media, **(c)** Laminar micelles

Table 5.3 Classification of association colloids

Type	Compound	Amphiphile	Genome
Anionic	Sodium lauryl sulphate	$CH_3(CH_2)_{11}OSO_3$	Na^+
Cationic	Cetyl trimethyl Ammonium bromide	$CH_3(CH_2)_{15}$ $N^+(CH_3)_{13}$	Br^-
Non ionic	Polyoxyethylene lauryl ether	$CH_3 (CH_2)_{10}$ CH_2O $(CH_2OCH_2)_2\ 3H$	-
Ampholytic	Dimethyl dodecyl ammonium propane sulfonate	$CH_3 (CH_2)_{11}$ $N^+(CH_3)_2 (CH_2)_3$ OSO_2	-

Mixtures of two or more amphiphiles are common. Assuming an ideal mixture, one can predict the CMC of the mixture from the CMC values of the pure amphiphiles and their mole fractions 'x' in the mixture, according to the equation.

$$\frac{1}{CMC} = \frac{x_1}{CMC_1} + \frac{x_2}{CMC_2}$$

The properties of Lyophilic, Lyophobic and association colloids are given in the Table 5.4.

Table 5.4 Comparison of properties of colloidal solution

Lyophilic	Association (Amphiphilic)	Lyophobic
1. Dispersed phase consists generally of large organic molecules lying within colloidal size range	Dispersed phase consists of aggregates (micelles) of small organic molecules or ions whose size individually is below colloidal range	Dispersed phase ordinarily consists of inorganic particles, such as gold or silver
2. Molecules of dispersed phase are solvated i.e., they are associated with the molecular comprising the dispersion medium	Hydrophilic or lipophilic portion of the molecules is solvated depending on whether the dispersion medium is aqueous or non-aqueous.	Little if an interaction occurs between particles and dispersion medium
3. Molecules disperse spontaneously to form colloidal solution	Colloidal aggregate are formed spontaneously when the concentration of amphiphiles exceeds the critical micelle concentration.	Material does not disperse spontaneously, and special procedures therefore must be adopted to produce colloidal dispersion

Table 5.4 *contd...*

Lyophilic	Association (Amphiphilic)	Lyophobic
4. Viscosity of the dispersion medium ordinarily is increased greatly by the presence of the dispersed phase; at sufficiently high concentrations, the solution may become a gel, viscosity and gel formation are related to saturation effects and to the shape of the molecules, which are usually highly asymmetric	Viscosity of the system increases as the concentration of the amphiphiles increases as micelles increase in number and become asymmetric	Viscosity of the dispersion medium is not greatly increased by the presence of lyophilic colloidal particles, which tend to be unsolvated and symmetric
5. Dispersions are stable generally in the presence of electrolyte, they may be salted out by high concentrations of very soluble electrolyte; effect is the primarily to degradation of lyophilic molecules	In aqueous solutions, the critical micelle concentration is reduced by the addition of electrolytes; salting out may occur at higher salt concentrations	Lyophilic dispersions are unstable in the presence of even small concentration of electrolytes; effect is due to neutralization of the charge on the particles; lyophilic colloids exert a protective effect.

5.5 Properties of Colloids

5.5.1 Optical Properties

The Faraday-Tyndall Effect

When a strong beam of light is passed through a colloidal solution, a visible cone, resulting from the scattering of light by the colloidal particles is formed. This is the faraday Tyndall effect.

Ultramicroscopy

Colloidal particles are too small to be seen with an optical microscope. Light scattering is employed in the ultramicroscope, first developed by Zsigmondy in which a cell containing the colloid is viewed against a dark background at right angles to an intense beam of incident light. The particles which exhibit Brownian motion, appears as spots of light against the dark background. The ultramicroscope is used in the technique of micro electrophoresis for measuring particle size.

Electron Microscopy

The electron microscope capable of giving actual pictures of the particles is used to observe the size, shape and structures of colloidal particle. The success of electron microscope is due to its high resolving power, defined is terms of d, the smallest distance by which two objects are separated get remain distinguishable. The smaller the wavelength of the radiation used, the smaller is d and the greater the resolving powers.

A microscope using visible light as its radiation source, gives a 'd' of about 0.2 μm. The radiation source of the electron microscope is a beam of high energy electrons having wave lengths in the region of 0.01 nm; 'd' is thus about 0.5 nm. The electron beams are focussed using electro magnet and the whole system is under a high vacuum of about 10^{-3}-10^{-5} Pa to give the electrons a free path.

A major disadvantage of electron microscope for viewing colloidal particles is that normally only dried samples can be examined. Consequently it is usually gives no information on solution or configuration in solution and the particles may be affected by sample preparation. A recent development which overcomes these problems is "Environmental scanning electron microscopy" (ESEM) which allows the observation of material in the wet state.

Light Scattering

When a beam of light is passed through a colloidal solution, some of the light may be absorbed, some is scattered and the remainder transmitted undisturbed through the sample. Due to the light scattered, the solution appears turbid, this is known as the "Tyndall effect". The turbidity of a solution is given by the expression.

$$I = I_0 \exp^{-1\tau}$$

where I_0 = intensity of the incident beam

I = intensity of transmitted light beam

l = length of the sample

τ = the turbidity.

Light scattering measurement is of great value for estimating particle size, shape and interactions, particularly of dissolved macro molecular materials as the turbidity depends on the size (mol. wt) of the colloidal material involved. As most colloids show very low turbidities, instead of measuring the transmitted light it is more convenient and accurate to measure the scattered light at an angle (usually 90°) relative to the incident beam.

The turbidity can be calculated from the intensity of the scattered light, provided the dimensions of the particle are small compared to the wavelength of the incident light by the expression

$$\tau = \frac{16\,\pi}{3}\ R_{90}$$

R_{90} – Raleigh ratio

The light scattering theory was modified by Debye and derived the following relationship between turbidity and molecular weight.

$$\frac{HC}{\tau} = \frac{1}{M} + 2BC \qquad\qquad ....(5.1)$$

where,

τ = turbidity (cm^{-1})

C = concentration of solute (g/cm^3) of solution

M = weight – average mol.wt in g/mole or Daltons

B = an interaction constant

H = constant for a particular system and is written as

$$H = \frac{32\,\pi^3\,n^2\,(dn/dc)^2}{3\,\lambda^4\,N} \qquad \qquad .....(5.2)$$

where,

n (dimensionless) = refractive index of the solution

c = concentration (g/cm^3)

λ = wavelength (cm^{-1})

$\dfrac{dn}{dc}$ = change in refractive index with concentration C.

N = Avogadro's number.

A part of HC/τ against concentration is result in a straight line with a scope of 2B. The intercept on the HC/τ axis is 1/M, the reciprocal of which yields the molecular weight of the colloid. The plot is given in Fig. 5.2.

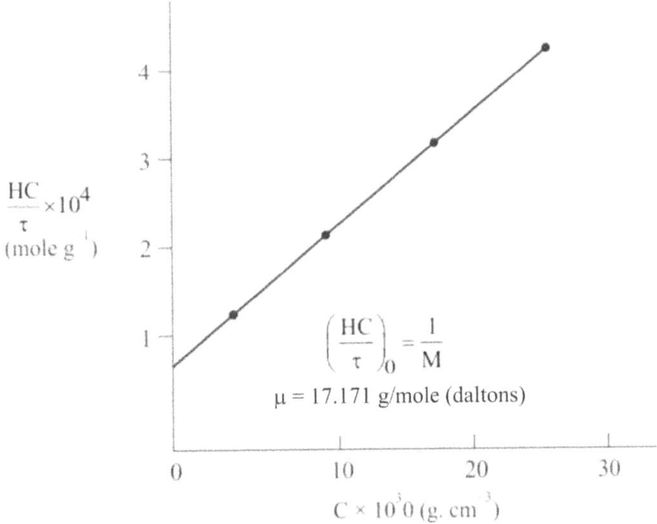

Fig. 5.2 A plot of $\dfrac{HC}{\tau}$ against the concentration of a polymer.

Light scattering measurement are particularly suitable for finding the size of the micelles of surface active agents and for the study of proteins and natural and synthetic polymers.

Light Scattering and Micelle Molecular Weight

When amphiphilic molecules associate to form micelles, the turbidity of the micellar dispersion differs from the turbidity of the solution of the amphiphilic molecules because micelles are now also percent in equilibrium with the monomeric species. Below the CMC, the concentration of monomers increases linearly with the total concentration, c; above the CMC, the monomer concentration remains linearly constant; i.e.,

$$C_{monomer} \cong CMC.$$

The concentration of micelles can therefore be written.

$$C_{micelle} = C - C_{monomer} \cong C - C_{CMC} \qquad \dots\dots(5.3)$$

The corresponding turbidity of the solution due to the presence of micelles is obtained by subtracting the turbidity due to monomers, $Y_{monomer} = Y_{CMC}$, from the total turbidity of the solution.

$$\tau_{micelle} = \tau - T_{CMC} \qquad \dots\dots(5.4)$$

Accordingly, equation 5.1 is modified to

$$\frac{H(C - C_{CMC})}{(\tau - \tau_{CMC})} = \frac{1}{M} + 2B\,(C - C_{CMC}) \qquad \dots\dots(5.5)$$

Subscript CMC indicates the turbidity of concentration at the critical micelle concentration.

B and H are the constants

M = molecular weight of micelle

M and B are obtained from the intercept and the slope respectively of a plot of $\dfrac{H(C - C_{CMC})}{(\tau - \tau_{CMC})}$ verses $(C - C_{CMC})$ in figure.

Equation (5.5) is valid for two component systems, i.e., for a micelle and a molecular surfactant in this instance.

5.5.2   Kinetic Properties of Colloids

In this section several properties of colloidal systems which relate to the motion of particles with respect to the dispersion medium will be considered. Thermal motion manifest itself in the form of Brownian motion diffusion and osmosis. Gravity (or a centrifugal fluid) leads to sedimentation. Viscous flow is the result of an externally applied force. Measurement of these properties enables molecular weights or particle size to be determined.

Brownian Motion

Colloidal particles are subject to random collisions with the molecules of dispersion medium with the result that each particle attains an irregular path. If the particles are observed under a microscope or the light scattered by colloidal particles is viewed using an ultramicroscope, an erratic motion is seen. This movement is referred to as Brownian motion.

Diffusion

As a result of Brownian motion, colloidal particles spontaneously diffuse from a region of higher concentration to one of lower concentration. The rate of diffusion is expressed by Fick's first law.

$$\frac{dm}{dt} = -DA\frac{dc}{dx} \qquad\qquad .....(5.6)$$

where, dm is the mass of substance diffusing in time dt across an area A under the influence of a concentration gradient dc/dx (minus sign denotes that diffusion takes place in the direction of decreasing concentration).

D is diffusion coefficient and has dimension of area per unit time. The diffusion coefficient of a dispersed material is related to the frictional coefficient f of the particles by Einstein's law of diffusion.

$$Df = k_B T \qquad\qquad .....(5.7)$$

k_B = Boltzmann constant

T = temperature

$\therefore$ The frictional coefficient is given by the Stoke's equation

$$f = 6\pi\eta a \qquad\qquad .....(5.8)$$

η = viscosity of the medium

a = the radius of the particle then

$$D = \frac{k_B T}{6\pi\eta a} = \frac{RT}{6\pi\eta a N_A} \qquad\qquad .....(5.9)$$

where, N_A = Avogadro constant

R = universal gas constant

$$K_B = \frac{R}{N_A}$$

The diffusion coefficient may be used to obtain the molecular weight of an approximately spherical particle, such as egg albumin and haemoglobin by using eq. 5.9 in the form:

$$D = \frac{RT}{6\pi\eta N_A} \sqrt[3]{\frac{4\pi N_A}{3M\bar{v}}} \qquad .....(5.10)$$

M = molecular weight

$\bar{v}$ = partial specific volume of the colloidal material.

Sedimentation

The sedimentation velocity (v) of spherical particles having a density ρ is a medium of density ρ_0 and a viscosity η_0 is given by stoke's law.

$$v = \frac{2r^2\,(\rho-\rho_0)g}{9\eta_0} \qquad .....(5.11)$$

g = acceleration due to gravity

If the particles are only subjected to the force of gravity then, due to Brownian motion, the lower size limit of particles obeying stoke's equation is about 0.5 μm. A stronger force than gravity is therefore needed for colloidal particles to sediment and this is done by using high speed centrifuge, termed as ultracentrifuge, which can produce a force of about 10^6g.

In a centrifuge g is replaces by w^2x, where w is the angular velocity and x is the distance of the particle from the centre of rotation and eq. (5.11) becomes

$$v = \frac{2r^2 g(\rho-\rho_0)w^2x}{9\eta_0} \qquad .....(5.12)$$

The ultracentrifuge is used in two distinct ways in investigating colloidal material.

In the *sedimentation velocity* method, a high centrifugal field is applied, upto about 44×10^5 g and the movement of the particles, monitored by changes in concentration, is measured at specific time intervals.

In the *sedimentation equilibrium* method, the colloidal material is subjected to much lower centrifugal field until sedimentation and diffusion tendencies balance one another an equilibrium distribution of particles throughout the sample is attained.

Sedimentation velocity: The velocity dx/dt of a particle in a unit centrifugal force can be expressed in terms of the svedberg coefficient is:

$$S = \frac{\dfrac{dx}{dt}}{w^2 x} \qquad ......(5.13)$$

Under the influence of centrifugal force, particles pass from portion x, at time t_1 to position x_2 at time t_2. The difference in concentration which can be measured by using changes in refractive index. Integration of eq. (5.13) using the above limits

$$S = \frac{ln\dfrac{x_2}{x_1}}{w^2\left(t_2 - t_1\right)} \qquad .....(5.14)$$

By suitable manipulation of equations 5.12, 5.13, 5.14 an expression giving mol. wt 'M' can be obtained

$$M = \frac{RT_s}{D\left(1 - \overline{v}\rho\right)} = \frac{RT\,ln\,{x_2}/{x_1}}{D\left(1 - \overline{v}\rho\right)\left(t_2 - t_1\right)w^2} \qquad .....(5.15)$$

where $\overline{v}$ is the partial specific volume of the particles combination of sedimentation and diffusion equation is made in the analysis giving

$$M = \frac{2RT\,ln\dfrac{C_2}{C_1}}{w^2\left(1 - \overline{v}\rho\right)\left(x_2^2 - x_1^2\right)} \qquad .....(5.16)$$

where C_1 and C_2 are the sedimentation equilibrium concentrations at distances x_1 and x_2 from the axis of rotation.

A disadvantage of the sedimentation equilibrium method is the length of time required to attain equilibrium is often as long as several days.

Osmotic Pressure

The osmotic pressure π of a dilute colloidal solution is described by the van't Hoff equation.

$$\pi = CRT \qquad .....(5.17)$$

Where, C is molar concentration of solution. This equation can be used to calculate the molecular weight of a colloidal in a dilute solution. Replacing C with c_g/M in eq. (5.17) in which C_g is the grams of solute per liter of solution.

M is the molecular weight, we get

$$\pi = \frac{C_g}{M} RT \qquad \qquad .....(5.18)$$

Then

$$\frac{\pi}{C_g} = \frac{RT}{M} \qquad \qquad .....(5.19)$$

which applies in a very dilute solution. The quantity π/C_g for a polymer having a molecular weight of say 50,000 is often a linear function of the concentration, C_g and the following equation can be written.

$$\frac{\pi}{C_g} = RT\left(\frac{1}{M} + BC_g\right) \qquad \qquad .....(5.20)$$

where, B is a constant for any particular solvent/solute system.

BC_g in eq. (5.20) is needed because eq. (5.19) holds only for ideal solutions i.e., only those containing low concentrations of sphero colloids.

Thus a plot of π/C versus C is linear with the value of intercept at $C \rightarrow 0\,C$ giving $\dfrac{RT}{M}$ enabling the molecular weight of the colloid to be calculated. The molecular weight obtained from osmotic pressure measurements is a number average value.

Viscosity

Viscosity is an expression of the resistance to flow of a system under an applied stress. An equation of flow applicable to colloidal dispersions of spherical particles was developed by Einstein

$$\eta = \eta_o \left(1 + 2.5\phi\right) \qquad \qquad .....(5.21)$$

where,

η_o = viscosity of the dispersion medium

η = viscosity of dispersion when the volume fraction of colloidal particles present in ϕ.

A number of viscosity coefficients may be defined with respect to above equation these include relative viscosity.

$$\eta_{rel} = \eta/\eta_o = 1 + 2.5\,\phi \qquad \qquad .....(5.22)$$

and specific viscosity

$$\eta_{SP} = \frac{\eta}{\eta_o} - 1 = \frac{(\eta - \eta_o)}{\eta_o} = 2.5\,\phi \qquad \qquad .....(5.23)$$

or
$$\frac{\eta_{SP}}{\phi} = 2.5$$

Since volume fraction is directly proportional to concentration, the eq. (5.23) can be written as

$$\frac{\eta_{SP}}{C} = k$$

where,

C = concentration expressed as grams of colloidal particles per 100 ms of total dispersion.

K = a constant

If η is determined for a number of concentrations of macromolecular material in solution and $\dfrac{\eta_{SP}}{C}$ is plotted against C then the intercept obtained on extrapolation of the linear plot to infinite dilution is known as the intrinsic viscosity (η). The plot is given in Fig. 5.3.

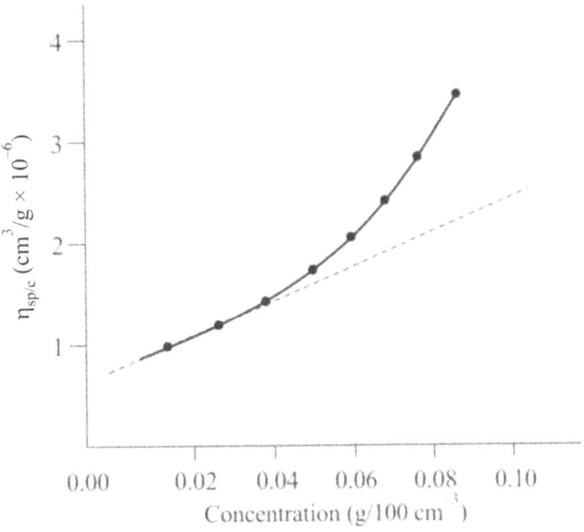

Fig. 5.3 Determination of molecular weight using viscosity data.

This constant may be used to calculate the molecular weight of the macromolecular material by making use of Mark-Houwink equation.

$$[\eta] = KM^a$$

where, K and a are constants characteristic of the particular polymer solvent system. These constants are obtained initially by determining (η) for a polymer fraction whose mol. wt has to be determined by another method such as sedimentation, osmotic pressure or light scattering.

5.5.3 Electrical Properties

The properties of colloids that depend on or are effected by the presence of a charge on the surface of a particle are discussed here.

Electrokinetic Phenomena

The movement of a charged surface with respect to an adjacent liquid phase is the basic principle underlying four electrokinetic phenomena; electrophoresis, electro osmosis, sedimentation potential and streaming potential.

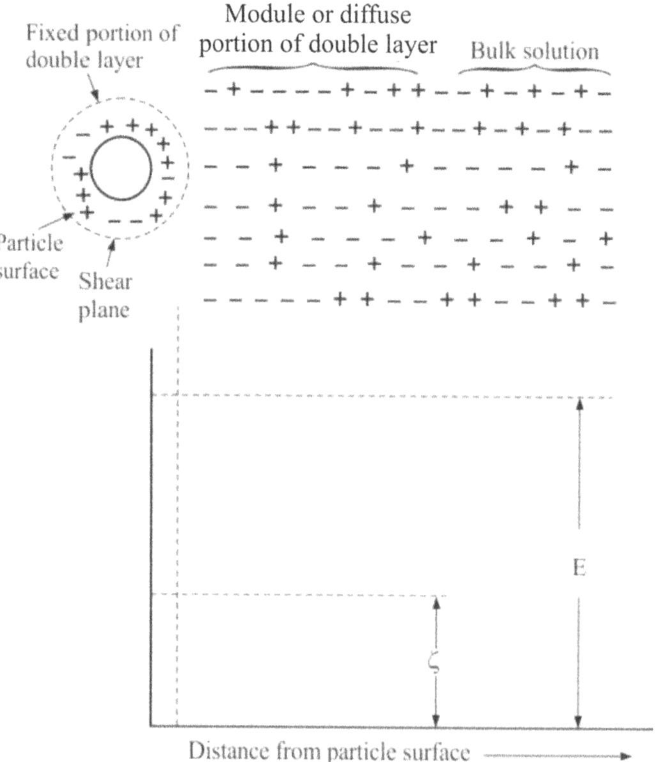

Fig. 5.4 Diffuse double layer and the zeta potential.

Electrophoresis involves the movement of a charged particle through a liquid under the influence of an applied potential difference. An electrophoresis cell fitted with two electrodes contains the dispersion. When a potential is applied across the electrodes, the particles migrate to oppositely charged electrode. It is given in Fig. 5.4. The rate of particle migration is observed by means of an ultramicroscope and is a function of the charge on the particle. Because the shear plane of the particle is located at the periphery of the tightly bound layer, the rate determining potential is the zeta potential. The relevant equation is

$$\zeta = \frac{v}{E} \times \frac{4\pi\eta}{\in} \times \left(9 \times 10^4\right)$$

ζ = zeta potential (in volts)

v = velocity of migration (cm/sec)

l = length of electrophoresis tube (in cm)

η = viscosity of the medium (in poises)

$\in$ = dielectric constant of the medium (volts/cm)

E = potential gradient (volts/cm)

The term $\dfrac{v}{\in}$ is known as the mobility.

Electroosmosis is essentially opposite to electrophoresis. In the latter, the application of a potential causes a charged particle to move relative to the liquid which is stationary. If the solid is rendered Immobile, (e.g., by forming a capillary or making the particles into a porous plug), however, the liquid now moves relative to the changed surface. This is electroosmosis, so called liquid moves through a plug or a membrane across when a potential is applied. The zeta potential can be obtained by determining the rate of flow of liquid through the plug under standard conditions.

Sedimentation Potential

Sedimentation potential, the reverse of electrophoresis, is the creation of a potential when particles undergo sedimentation. E.g., a glass tube or packed powder bid streaming potential: differs from electroosmosis in that the potential is created by forcing a liquid to flow through a plug or bed of particles. E.g., a glass tube, by an applied electric field.

Whereas the technique of micro electrophoresis finds application in the measurement of zeta potentials.

To test colloid stability e.g.: polystyrene latex dispersions

To test stability of coarse dispersions e.g.: suspensions and emulsions.

In identification of charge and other surface characteristics of water insoluble drugs and cells such as blood and bacteria.

Donnan Membrane Equilibrium

If sodium chloride is placed in solution on one side of a semipermeable membrane and a negatively charged colloid together with its concentrations R^-Na^+ is placed on the other side, the sodium and chloride ions can pass freely across the barrier but not the colloidal anionic particles. In the system R^- is the non-diffusible colloidal anion and vertical line separating the various species represents the semipermeable membrane. The volumes of solution on the two sides of the membrane are considered to be equal.

Outside (o)	inside (i)
Na^+	Na^+
Cl^-	Cl^-

After equilibrium has been established, the concentration in dilute solutions of sodium chloride must be the same on both sides of the membrane, according to the principle of escaping tendencies.

$$\therefore \quad [Na^+]_o\,[Cl^-]_o = [Na^+];\,[Cl^-]\,i \qquad .....(5.24)$$

The condition of electroneutrality must also apply that is, the concentration of positively charged ions in the solutions on either side of the membrane must balance the concentration of negatively charged ions. Therefore, on the outside,

$$[Na^+]_o = [Cl^-]_o \qquad .....(5.25)$$

and inside,

$$[Na^+]_i = [R^-]_i + [Cl^-]_i \qquad .....(5.26)$$

Equations (5.25) and (5.26) are substituted in (1)

$$[Cl^-]_o^{\,2} = ([Cl^-]_i + [R^-]_i)\,[Cl^-]i = \left[Cl^-\right]_i^2 \left(1 + \frac{\left[R^-\right]i}{\left[Cl^-\right]i}\right) \quad .....(5.27)$$

$$\frac{\left[Cl^-\right]_o}{\left[Cl^-\right]i} = \sqrt{1 + \frac{\left[R^-\right]i}{\left[Cl^-\right]i}} \qquad .....(5.28)$$

Eq. (5.28), the donnan membrane equilibrium gives the ratio of concentrations of the diffusible anion outside and inside the membrane at equilibrium. The equation shows that a negatively charged polyelectrolyte inside a semipermeable sac would influence the equilibrium concentration ratio of a diffusible anion. It tends to drive the ion of the charge out through the membrane.

When $[R^-]i$ is large compared with $[Cl^-]i$ the ratio roughly equals $\sqrt{\left[R^-\right]i}$, if $[Cl^-]i$ is quite large with respect to $[R^-]i$, the ratio becomes equal to unity, and the concentration of the salt is thus equal on both sides of the membrane. If $[Cl^-]$ in equation (5.28) is replaced by the concentration of the diffusible drug, anion at [D⁻] at equilibrium and [R⁻] is used to represent the concentration of polyelectrolyte at equilibrium then the equation becomes

$$\frac{\left[D^-\right]_o}{\left[D^-\right]_i} = \sqrt{1 + \frac{\left[R^-\right]_i}{\left[D^-\right]_i}} \qquad\qquad .....(5.29)$$

5.6 Solubilisation

The property of surface active agents to cause an increase in the solubility of organic compounds in aqueous system is called solubilisation. This property is observed only at and above the CMC, thus indicating that the micelles are involved in the phenomenon. In general, the increased solubility of the solubilised material (solubilisate) can be explained in terms of partition between the aqueous phase and the hydrocarbon interior of the micelles or by adsorption at the micellar surface. Thus it is believed that non-polar hydrocarbons are taken into solution in the interior of the micelles, and polar water soluble compounds such as sugar and glycerol are absorbed at the micelle/water interface as shown in (a) and (b) in Fig. (5.5). Compounds with amphipathic character, such as octonol and phenol, are believed to become oriented in the palisade layer in a similar manner to the surface active agent, i.e., with their polar groups directed towards the aqueous phase and their lipophilic groups inside the micelle as shown at (c) in Fig. (5.5). A possible additional mechanism for the effect of non-ionic micelles on the solubility of certain compounds e.g.: Phenol involves inclusion of these compounds between the long hydrophilic polyoxy ethylene chains as shown at (d) in Fig. (5.5).

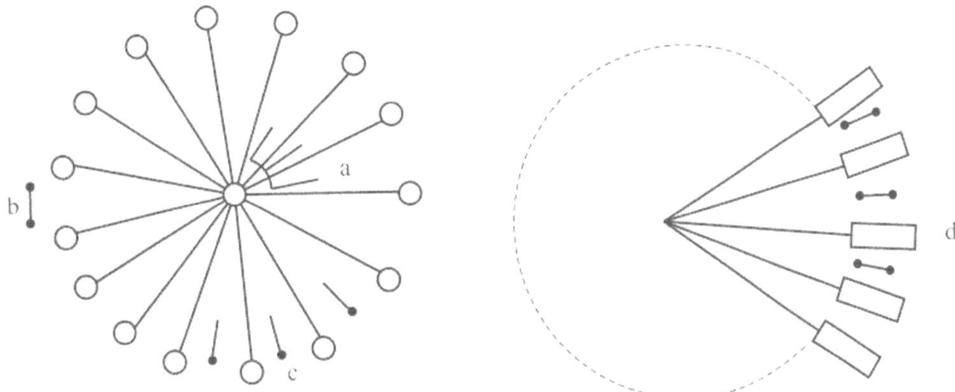

Fig.5.5 Solubilisation within micelles

(a) non-polar tail, **(b)** polar lead, **(c)** Amphipathic molecules oriented in palisade layer, **(d)** Polar molecules oriented between polyoxy ethylene chains of a non-ionic surface active agent

CMCs may be determined by solubilisation measurements preferably using a solid dye stuff that is virtually insoluble in water. The amount of dye stuff in solution remains reasonably constant until the CMC of the surface active agent is reached and then increases rapidly. Dyes are commonly used in such determinations because of the ease of analysis of the solutions by optical methods. The advantage of this method includes long periods of stirring necessary to ensure that equilibrium conditions have been reached.

5.6.1 Factors Affecting Solubilization

A. Molecular Structure of the Surface Active Agent

1. Hydro Carbon Chain

(a) *Chain length*: An increase in the hydrocarbon chain length causes a logarithmic decrease in the CMC at constant temperature as shown by eq (5.30).

$$\log C = A - B_m \qquad\qquad .....(5.30)$$

where, C is the CMC, m is the number of carbon atoms in the chain, A and B are constants for a homologous series of compounds.

(b) *Branched Hydrocarbon chains*: Branching of a hydrocarbon chain causes an increase in CMC since the decrease in free energy arising from the aggregation of branched chain molecules is less than that obtained with the value for the analogous saturated compound.

(c) *Unsaturation*: The CMC is increased by about three to four times by the presence of one double bond when compared with the value for the analogous saturated compound.

2. The Hydrophilic Group

(a) *Type of Hydrophilic Group*: The value of the constant A in eq. (5.30) varies with the type of hydrophilic group common to each homologous series. However, the effect of different ionic groups on the CMC is small, provided complete ionic dissociation occurs, because the amount of work necessary to overcome the electrical repulsion between the ions of same charge is similar.

(b) *Number of Hydrophilic Groups*: The electrical repulsive force between adjacent ions in a micelle increases at the no. of ionic groups increases. Increase in no. of hydrophilic group increases the solubility of the surface active agent. Both these effects will lead to an increase in the CMC.

(c) *Position of Hydrophilic Group:* The CMC tends to increase as the polar group is moved from the terminal position towards the middle of the hydrocarbon chain.

B. Effect of Addition

1. *Simple Electrolytes*: The CMC decreases on addition of salts. The most important factors concerned in the overall effect are the concentration and no. of charges on the ions of opposite charge (gegenious) to that carried by that micelle. The effect of these factors is given by eq. (5.31).

$$ln \; c = -k. \; ln \; c_1 + constant \qquad \qquad .....(5.31)$$

k = a constant with a value of 0.4 app

c = CMC

c_1 = total gegerion concentration

For surface active acute with two ionic groups eq. (5.31) becomes.

$$ln c = -2k \; . \; ln c_1 + constant \qquad \qquad .....(5.32)$$

2. *Other Surface Active Agents*: The CMCs of mixtures of surface active agents appear to vary between the limiting values of the highest and lowest CMCs of the individual components.

3. *Alcohol*: CMCs are decreased by the addition of alcohol.

4. *Hydrocarbons*: Solubilization of hydrocarbons causes an increase in micellar size, which results in an increase in the radius of curvature of the micellar surface which may cause a slight separation of adjacent ions and therefore, a decrease in the repulsive forces.

CHAPTER 6

MICROMERITICS

6.1 Introduction

The science and technology of small particles was denoted as micromeritics. Knowledge and control of the size and the size range of particles are of profound importance in pharmacy. Thus size and surface area of a particle can be related in a significant way to the physical, chemical and pharmacologic properties of a drug. 'Colloidal Dispersions' are characterized by particles that are too small to be seen in the ordinary microscope. The unit of particle size used most frequently in micromeritics is the micrometer, μm also called as micro 'μ' and it is equal to 10^{-6} m, 10^{-4} cm and 10^{-3} mm.

6.1.1 Significance of Particle size in various Dosage Forms

The properties of powder can be influenced directly by size of particles or indirectly by the surface area of powder which is dependent on size.

Suspensions: when the powders are suspended in liquids the behaviour and flow properties will depend on the particle size. If particles are small, solid clay like sediment will form as the solids settle out, and it is very difficult to redisperse. On the other hand, large particles, although redispersed easily, will settle rapidly and make the suspension difficult to use. Therefore "optimum" particle size is needed for any suspension.

Mixture of Solids: particle size has a great effect on the mixing of solid substances and on the stability of mixture.

Solid/Fluid Separation: Processes for separating solids from fluids such as filtration and sedimentation are influenced greatly by particle size.

Granule Size in Tablets: Successful tablet manufacture requires careful control of the size of granules from which the tablets are compressed.

Process Factors: Particle size effects the flow characters of a powder during the manufacture of a product.

6.1.2 Significance of Particle Surface Area

As the particle size decreases, the surface area of the particle increases.

108

Mass Transfer Process: This means that operations such as solution, extraction, drying will be influenced indirectly by particle surface area.

Adsorption: Adsorption is the surface phenomenon. This means that the adsorptive capacity of a material will increase as particle surface area increases.

Absorption of Drugs: Absorption of a drug will depend on the particle surface area.

6.1.3 Particle and Size Distribution

In a collection of particles of more than one size, two properties are important namely:

(a)   The shape and surface area of the individual particles and

(b)   The size range and number or weight of particles present

The size of a sphere is readily expressed in terms of its diameter. As the degree of asymmetry of particle increases, it is difficult to express the size in terms of meaningful diameter.

Equivalent Spherical Diameter: It relates the size of the particle to the diameter of a sphere having the same surface area, volume or diameter. Thus the surface diameter (ds) is the diameter of a sphere having the same surface area as the particle in question. The diameter of a sphere having the same volume as the particle is the volume diameter (dv). The projected diameter (dp) is the diameter of a sphere having the same observed area as the particle when viewed normal to its most stable plane.

The size can also be expressed as the stokes diameter (d_{st}) which describes an equivalent sphere undergoing sedimentation as the same rate as the asymmetric particle.

The projected diameter is obtained by microscopic techniques, whereas the stokes diameter is determined from sedimentation studies on the suspended particles.

Average Particle Size: Suppose we have conducted a microscopic examination of a sample of a powder and recorded the number of particles lying within various size ranges. To compare these values with those from, say, a second batch of the same material, we usually compute an average or mean diameter as our basis for comparison.

'Edmundson' derived a general equation for the average particle size, whether it be an arithmetic, a geometric or a harmonic mean diameter.

$$d_{mean} = \left(\frac{\sum nd^{P+f}}{\sum nd^f} \right)^{1/p} \qquad \qquad .....(6.1)$$

Here 'n' is the number of particles in a size range 'd' is the midpoint, that is one of the equivalent diameters, 'P' is an index related to the size of an individual particle.

The value of the index 'P' also describes whether the mean is arithmetic ('P' is positive), geometric (P is zero), or harmonic ('P' is negative)

nd^f is the frequency with which a particle in a certain size range occurs.

'f' is the frequency index and it has values of 0, 1, 2 (or) 3.

The size of frequency distribution is expressed in terms of the total number, length, surface or volume of the particles respectively.

6.1.4 Particle-Size Distribution

As the dimensions of particles increase, the particles change their nature and the forces acting on them change. Fine powder particles less than 100 μm in diameter are governed by surface forces and particles about 100 mm in diameter are governed by gravitational forces. Frequency distribution curve is obtained when the number or weight of particles lying within a certain size range is plotted against the mean particle size. Size-frequency distribution is represented in Fig. (6.1).

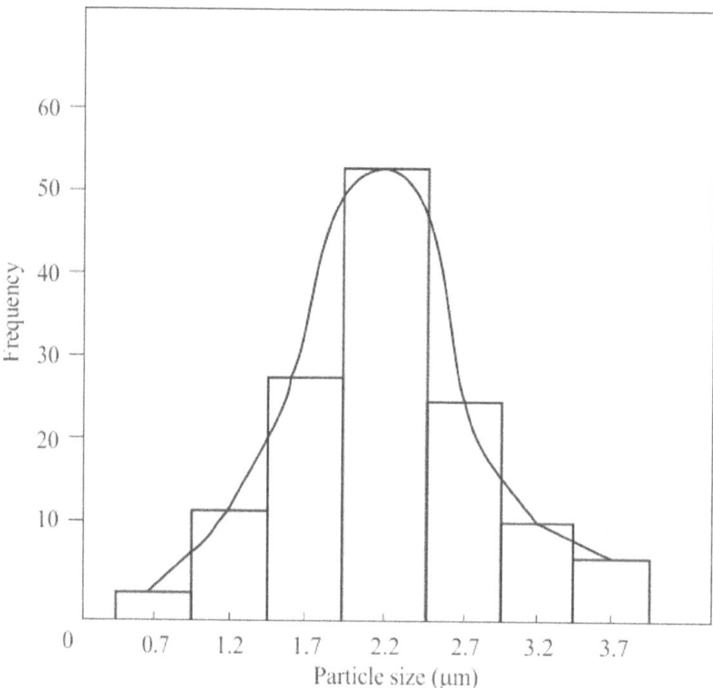

Fig. 6.1 Representing size-frequency distribution.

If the particle occurs more frequently in a sample it is called as mode.

Standard deviation 'σ' is an indication of the distribution about the mean.

6.1.5 Number and Weight Distribution

Number distribution implying that they were collected by a counting technique such as microscopy. Frequently, we are interested in obtaining data based on a weight, rather than a number, distribution.

Although it can be achieved by using a technique such as sedimentation (or sieving, it will be more convenient, if the number data are already at hand, to convert the number distribution to a weight distribution and vice versa. Fig. 6.2 (a) and (b) represents number and weight distribution.

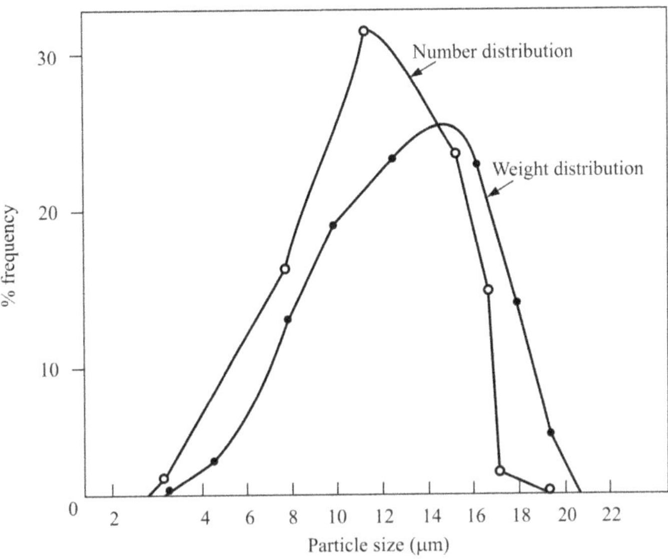

Fig. 6.2(a) Representing number and weight distribution.

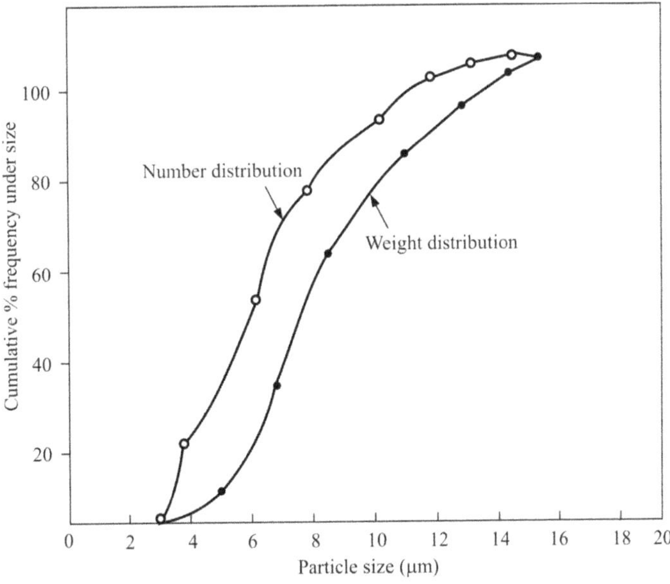

Fig. 6.2(b) Representing number and weight distribution.

6.2 Methods for Determining Particle Size

Many methods are available for deter mining particle size. Microscopy, sieving, sedimentation, and the determination of particle volume are discussed in the following section.

6.2.1 Optical Microscopy

It should be possible to use ordinary microscope for particle size measurement in the range of 0.2 to about 100 µm. According to the microscopic method an emulsion or suspension, diluted or undiluted is mounted on a slide and placed on mechanical stage. The microscope eye piece is fitted with a micrometer by which the size of the particles can be estimated. The field can be projected on to a screen where the particles are measured more easily, or a photograph can be taken from which a slide is prepared and projected on a screen for measurement.

The particles are measured along an arbitrarily chosen fixed line, generally made horizontally across the centre of particle. Popular measurements are the 'Feret diameter', 'Martin diameter' and the Projected area diameter, all of which can be defined by reference to Fig. 6.3 'Martin diameter' is the length of a line that bisects the particle image. The line can be drawn in any direction but must be in the same direction for all particles measured. Martin diameter is identified by the number 1 in Fig. 6.3. 'Feret diameter' corresponding to the number 2 in Fig. 6.3, is the distance between two tangents on opposite sides of the particle parallel to some fixed direction, the 'Y' direction in the Fig. 6.3. The third measurement, number 3 in Fig. (6.3) is the 'Projected area diameter'. It is the diameter of a circle with the same area as that of the particle observed perpendicular to the surface on which the particle rests. Electronic scanners have been developed to remove the necessity of measuring particles by visual observation.

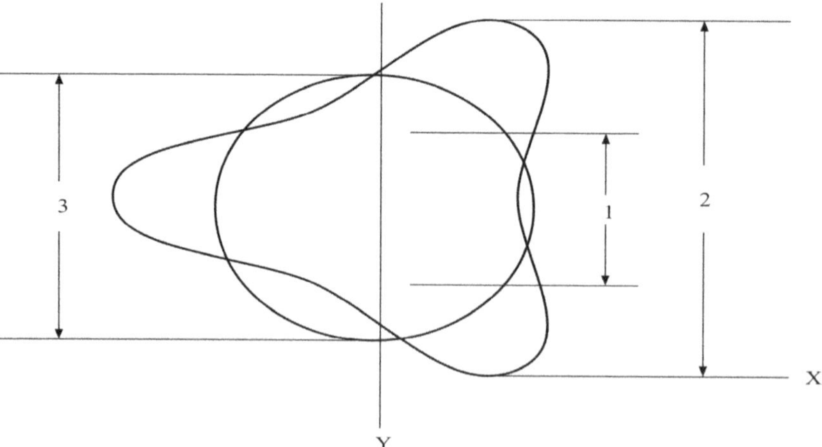

Fig. 6.3 A general diagram providing definitions of Feret, Martin, and projected diameters.

The disadvantage of the microscopic method is that the diameter is obtained from only two dimensions of the particle length and breadth, No estimation of the depth of the particle is ordinarily available.

6.2.2 Sieving

Sieves are generally used for grading coarser particles, by the extreme care they also employed for screening material as fine as 44 μm. Sieves produced by photo etching and electroforming techniques are available with apertures from 90 μm to as low as 5 μm. For testing of powders a mass of sample is placed on the proper sieve in a mechanical shaker. The powder is shaken for a definite period of time and the material that passes through one sieve and is retained on the next finer sieve is collected and weighed.

Another approach is to assign the particles on the lower sieve the arithmetic or geometric mean size of the two screens.

When a detailed analysis is desired, the sieves can be arranged in a nest of about five with the coarsest at the top. A carefully weighed sample of powder is placed on the top sieve, and after the sieves are shaken for a predetermined period of time, the powder retained on each sieve is weighed.

6.2.3 Sedimentation Method

These are based on the measurement of the rate at which particles of the powder settled out from a liquid in which they have been dispersed. The technique is widely employed and extended to sizes of about 0.5 μm under special circumstances by using a centrifuge to accelerate the settlement. In the incremental method the powder is suitably dispersed in the liquid contained in a tall vessel. 10 ml samples are withdrawn at predetermined times from a known depth below the surface and the weight of powder present in each sample is determined either by evaporating the liquid and weighing the residue.

In order to calculate the range of particle sizes present in each sample, stoke's law is used. This applies strictly only to dilute dispersions where the concentration of solid is less than 2% w/w.

This can be written as

$$V = \frac{h}{t} = \frac{d^2\left(\rho - \rho'\right)g}{18\eta} \qquad \text{....(6.2)}$$

where,

V = velocity of fall of a particle

h = depth in cm below the surface from which sample is withdrawn after t seconds

d = diameter of the particle in cm

ρ = density of material in gm/ml

ρ' = the density of liquid in gm/ml

g = gravitational constant 98/cm s^{-2}

η = viscosity of liquid in poises.

For applying stoke's law, a further requirement is that the flow of dispersion medium around the particle as it sediments is laminar or stream line. Whether the flow is turbulent or is laminar or stream line. Whether the flow is turbulent or laminar is indicated by dimensionless Reynolds number R_e

$$R_e = \frac{vd\rho_o}{\eta_o} \qquad ....(6.3)$$

Rearranging equation eq. (6.3) with eq. (6.2)

$$V = \frac{R_e \eta}{d\rho_o} = \frac{d^2(\rho_s - \rho_o)g}{18\eta} \qquad .....(6.4)$$

thus

$$d^3 = \frac{18R_e\eta^2}{(\rho_s - \rho_o)\rho_o g} \qquad .....(6.5)$$

Stoke's law cannot be used if R_e is greater than 0.2 because turbulence appears at this value.

Pipette method is used because of ease of analysis, accuracy and economy of equipment.

The Andreasen apparatus (Fig. 6.4) usually consists of a 550 ml vessel containing 10 ml pipette sealed into a ground glass stopper. When the pipette is placed in the cylinder, its lower tip is 20 cm below the surface of suspension a 1% or 2% suspension of the particles in a medium containing a suitable deflocculating agent is introduced into the vessel and brought to the 550 ml mark. The stoppered vessel is shaken to distribute the particles uniformly. At various time intervals 10 ml samples were withdrawn and discharged by means of two-way stopcock. The samples are evaporated and weighed. The particle diameter corresponding to various time periods is calculated from stoke's law. The residue or dried sample obtained at a particular time is the weight fraction having particles of size less than size obtained by stoke's law calculation for that time period of settling. The weight of each sample residue is therefore called the weight underside and the sum of successive weights is cumulative weight undersize.

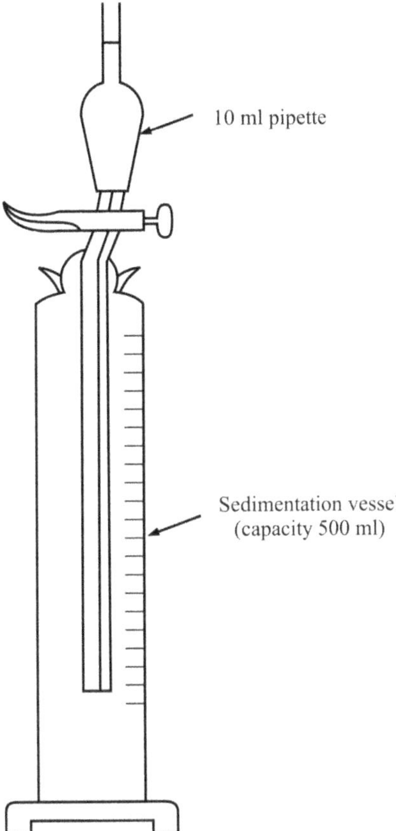

Fig. 6.4 Andreasen apparatus.

6.2.4 Particle Volume Measurement

A popular instrument for measuring the volume of particles is the Coulter Counter. This instrument operates on the principle that when a particle suspended in a conducting liquid passes through a small orifice on either side of which are electrodes, a change in electric resistance occurs.

This apparatus is coming increasingly into use in pharmacy for determining the particle size powders (Edmundson 1967) and depends on the ability to prepare a suspension of the sample free from floccules. The suspension is made up in a suitable electrolyte solution e.g., NaCl, and is then drawn through small orifice having an electrode on each side. As such particle passes through, it displaces its own volume of electrolyte within orifice and increases its electrical resistance. The resulting voltage pulses are proportional to the particle volume; they are amplified, scaled and counted and yield a particle size distribution curve extending under ideal circumstances, down to about 0.2 μm.

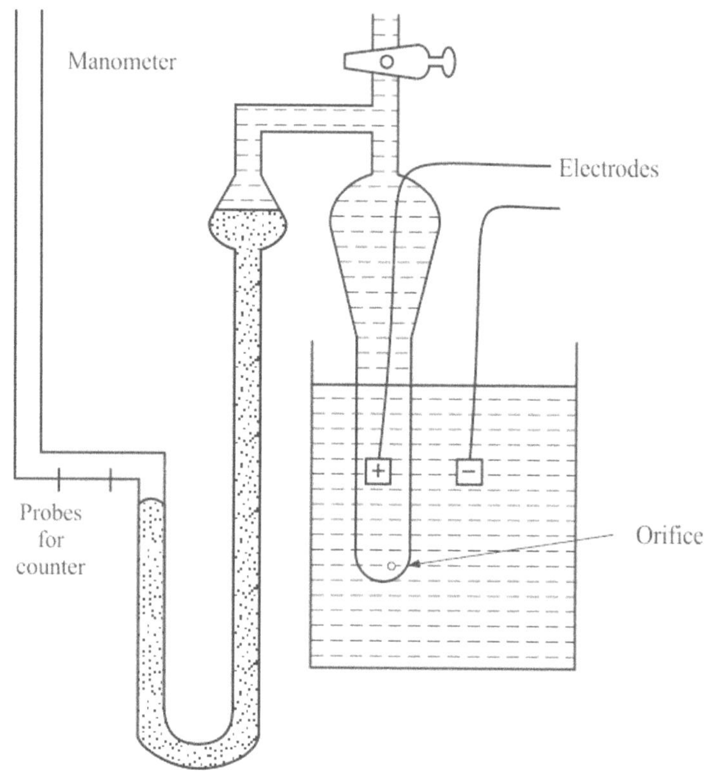

Fig. 6.5 Coulter counter approach.

6.3 Particle Shape and Surface Area

The shape of a particle effects the flow and packing properties of a powder.

6.3.1 Particle Shape

The more asymmetric of a particle the greater is the surface area per unit volume. Surface area or volume of a sphere because for such particle

$$\text{Surface area} = \pi d^2 \qquad \qquad .....(6.6)$$

$$\text{and} \qquad \text{volume} = \frac{\pi d^3}{6} \qquad \qquad .....(6.7)$$

where, d = diameter of a particle

Specific Surface

The specific surface is the surface area per unit volume S_v; or per unit weight S_w.

$$S_v = \frac{\text{Surface area of Particle}}{\text{Volume of Particles}} \qquad \qquad .....(6.8)$$

$$S_w = \frac{S_v}{\rho} \qquad \qquad .....(6.9)$$

where, ρ = true density of particles.

6.3.2 Methods for Determining Surface Area

Two methods are commonly available for calculating surface area. They are adsorption method and air permeability method. In the first, the amount of a gas or liquid solute that is adsorbed onto the sample of powder to form a monolayer is a direct function of surface area of sample. The second method depends on the fact that the rate at which gas or liquid permeates a bed of powder is related.

Gas Adsorption Method

The amount of gas that will be adsorbed by a powder also provides a means of determining its total surface area, and this type of measurement is conveniently carried out with the Perkin-Elmer shell Sorptometer. Basically the apparatus consists of two valves for controlling the flow of nitrogen and helium gas. These flow through a cold trap then through the reference arm of a detector unit, then through an adsorption tube containing a known weight of sample which has previously been freed from adsorbed gas by subjecting it to a high vacuum and finally through the measuring arm of detector.

The amount of nitrogen adsorbed by the powder at series of different partial pressures of nitrogen is obtained by continually measuring the thermal conductivity of the emergent gas stream, and the surface area per gram of the sample is then obtained by BET equation.

Gas Permeability Method

The gas permeability of a powder provides a measure of its surface area and if it is assumed that the particles are all of equal size and in spherical shape, then their mean diameter can be evaluated.

In the Lea and Nurse method dry air is forced at constant pressure through a bed of powder under investigation. In the Rigden method, which has been adopted from it, air is allowed to escape from a reservoir through the powder bed and the time for the pressure to fall from one specified level to another is measured.

In Rigder apparatus two ends of the cell E containing the powder are connected to the two ends of a 'U' tube containing non volatile oil. The equilibrium level of the oil is at 'C'. The oil is sucked into one arm Y of the manometer by meant of bulb F and as it returns to the equilibrium level, it forces air through powder bed. The time taken for a given volume of oil to travel between starting line to mark A or B on the manometer is measured and the specific surface is calculated from Kozeny equation.

$$S = \left[\frac{\varepsilon^3}{(1-\varepsilon)^2} \frac{A}{5\eta L} \frac{\beta pg}{V} ln\left(\frac{h_2}{h_1}\right) \frac{t}{d^2} \right]^{1.3} \qquad .....(6.10)$$

where

S = specific surface in $cm^2 g^{-1}$

ε = porosity

A = cross sectional area of powder bed

η = gas viscosity in poises

L = length of powder bed

β = atmospheric pressure in cm of liquid of density ρ gcm^{-3}

g = gravitational constant in cms^{-2}

V = volume of reservoir

h_2 = final reservoir pressure in cm of liquid

h_1 = initial reservoir pressure in cm of liquid

d = density of powder sample in gcm^{-3}

t = time in seconds for air pressure to fall from h_1 to h_2

6.4   Derived Properties of Powders

6.4.1 Porosity

A powder such as zinc oxide is placed in a graduated cylinder and total volume is noted. The volume occupied is known as bulk volume V_b. If the powder is non porous, that is has no internal pores, the bulk volume of the powder consists of the true volume of the solid particles plus the volume of the spaces between the particles. The volume of the spaces, known as void volume 'v' is given by equation.

$$V = V_b - V_P \qquad .....(6.11)$$

In which V_p is true volume of particles.

The porosity 'ε' of the powder is defined as the ratio of the void volume to the bulk volume of the packing.

$$\varepsilon = \frac{V_b - V_P}{V_b} = 1 - \frac{V_P}{V_b} \qquad \qquad .....(6.12)$$

6.4.2 Packing Arrangements

Two packing arrangements are seen in powder beds

    (a)   Closest or rhombohedra

    (b)   Most open, loosest or cubic packing

The particles in real powders are neither spherical in shape nor uniform in size. Most powders in practice have porosities between 30% and 50%.

Densities of Particles

Density is universally defined as weight per unit volume; for convenience three types of densities can be defined:

    (a)   The true density of the material itself, exclusive of voids and intraparticle pores larger than molecular dimensions in crystal lattice.

    (b)   Granule density is determined by displacement of mercury, which does not penetrate at ordinary pressures into pores smaller than about 10 μm.

    (c)   The bulk density as determined from the bulk volume and the weight of a dry powder in a graduated cylinder.

True density ρ, is the density of actual solid material. Methods for determining the density of non porous solids by displacement in liquids in which they are insoluble. If the material is porous, true density can be determined by use of helium densiometer. The volume of the empty apparatus is first determined by introducing a known quantity of helium. A weighed amount of powder is then introduced into the sample tube, adsorbed gases are removed from powder by an outgassing procedure; and helium which is not adsorbed by the material is again introduced. The procedure is read on a mercury manometer and by the application of gas laws, the volume of helium surrounding particles and penetrating into small cracks and pores is calculated. The difference between the volume of helium filling the empty apparatus and the volume of helium in presence of powder sample yields the volume occupied by powder. Knowledging the weight of powder, one is then able to calculate true density.

Granule density ρg, can be determined by a method similar to liquid displacement method. Mercury is used because it fills the void spaces but fails to penetrate into internal pores of the particles. The volume of the particles together with their intraparticle spaces then gives granular volume, and from a knowledge of powder weight one finds the granule density.

The intraparticle porosity of granules can be computed from a knowledge of true and granule density. The porosity is given by equation

$$\in_{intraparticle} = \frac{V_g - V_\rho}{V_g} = 1 - \frac{V_\rho}{V_g} = 1 - \frac{weight/true\ density}{weight/granule\ density} \qquad .....(6.13)$$

or $\qquad \in_{intraparticle} = 1 - \dfrac{Granule\ density}{True\ density} \qquad\qquad .....(6.14)$

Bulk density P_b is defined as the mass of a powder divided by the bulk volume. A sample of about 50 cm^3 of powder that has previously been passed through a U.S standard No.20 sieve is carefully introduced into a 100 ml graduated cylinder. The cylinder is dropped at 2-sec intervals onto a hard wood surface three times from a height of 1 inch. The bulk density is obtained by dividing the weight of the sample in grams by the final volume in cm^3 of the sample contained in cylinder. The bulk density does not actually reach a maximum until the container has been dropped or tapped some 500 times.

The inter space or void porosity of a powder of porous granules is the relative volume of interspace voids to the bulk volume of powder, exclusive of intraparticle pores. The bulk density and granule density is expressed by equation

$$\in_{interspace} = \frac{V_b - V_g}{V_b} = 1 - \frac{V_g}{V_b} = 1 - \frac{weight/Granule\ density}{weight/Bulk\ density} \qquad .....(6.15)$$

The total porosity of a porous powder is made up of voids between the particles as well as pores within the particles.

The total porosity is defined as

$$\in_{total} = \frac{V_b - V_p}{V_b} = 1 - \frac{V_P}{V_b} \qquad\qquad .....(6.16)$$

6.4.3 Bulkiness

The reciprocal of bulk density is often called bulkiness. Bulkiness increases with a decrease in particle size.

6.4.4 Angle of Repose

The frictional forces in a loose powder can be measured by the angle of repose ϕ. This is the maximum angle possible between the surface of a pile of powder and the horizontal plane. If more material is added to the pile, it slides down the slides until the mutual friction of the particles, producing a surface at an angle ϕ, is in equilibrium with the gravitational force. The tangent of the angle of repose is equal to the coefficient of friction 'μ'.

$$\tan\phi = \mu \qquad\qquad .....(6.17)$$

CHAPTER 7

RHEOLOGY

7.1 Introduction

The term Rheology was derived from Greek, Rheo means "to flow" and Logos means "science". It was suggested by Bingham & Crawford to describe the flow of liquids and deformation of solids.

Rheology is the branch of science that deals with deformation, including flow of matter (or) it is the science concerned with deformation of matter under the influence of stress (force per unit area) which may be applied perpendicularly to the surface of a body (a tensile stress), tangentially to the surface (a shearing stress) or at any angle to the surface.

Deformations are of two types:

1. Spontaneously reversible/Elastic deformations – work used in deformation is recoverable.
2. Permanent or irreversible deformations exhibited by viscous bodies – the work used in deformation production is dissipated as heat and not recoverable.

In the former case, the body regain its original state after removing the stress where as in later case, the deformation in body may not recover completely when stress is removed.

The term "Strain" is used to indicate the deformation of a solid, where in case of fluid "Rate of Shear" is used since it undergoes flow when stress is applied.

Viscosity of a fluid may be described as index of resistance to flow/movement of fluids.

The higher the viscosity, the greater is the resistance to flow.

7.1.1 Importance

It is essential to understand rheological properties of pharmaceutical materials, to prepare, to evaluate, to develop and in performance of pharmaceutical dosage forms.

121

1. Rheology is involved in mixing and flow of materials, packing of materials into their containers and their removal prior to use i.e., pouring from a bottle, exhaustion from a tube or passing through a syringe needle.

2. The rheological property of a particular product can effect its patient acceptability, physical stability and even biological availability/bioavailability.

3. It helps in characterizing and classifying fluids and semi-solids.

4. The rheological principles govern the circulation of blood and lymph through capillaries and large blood vessels, mucus flow, transition of luminal content through GIT, muscle contraction, bones bending, cartilage stretching etc.

5. The fluidity of solution which are administered through I.V., strength of surfaces and ligatures are important rheological properties.

6. The rheological phenomenon is also involved in spreading lotion on skin, spraying liquids from atomizers or aerosols, in mechanical properties of glass or plastic or glass containers of rubber/polymeric closures.

7. This property also controls and modulates the drug release from dosage forms and delivery systems (in formulation matrix).

7.1.2 Classification

According to type of flow, there are 2 types of systems.

1. Newtonian system
2. Non-Newtonian system

Simple fluids which follows Newton's law are called Newtonian and which doesn't follows/obey Newton's law are called Non-newtonian fluids.

Note: *Newton's law:* Direct proportionality between shear stress and Rate of shear. (or)

Rate of flow is directly proportional to applied stress.

7.2   Newtonian System/Fluids

Newtonian liquids are preferred with solutions of lower molecular weight compounds.

7.2.1 Newton's Law of Flow

A "block" of liquid is considered, which consists of parallel plates of molecules, similar to deck of cards. It is shown in Fig.7.1. Assume as if the bottom layer is fixed/stationary. When a tangential force is applied to uppermost plate, that each subsequent layer will move at progressively decreasing velocity. The difference of velocity (dv) between two plates/planes of liquid which are separated by an infinitesimal distance (dr) is the velocity gradient or rate of shear.

$$\text{Rate of shear (G)} = \frac{dv}{dr} \qquad \qquad .....(7.1)$$

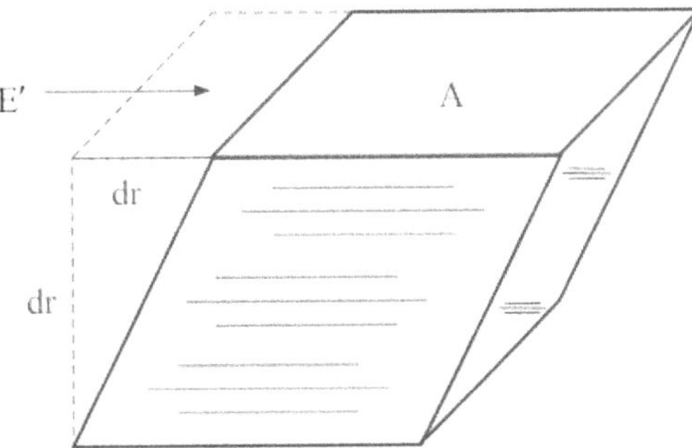

Fig. 7.1 Representation of the shearing force required to produce a definite velocity gradient between the parallel planes of a block of material.

The stress, which is force per unit area required to bring flow is shearing stress.

$$\text{Shearing stress, } (F) = \frac{F'}{A} \qquad \qquad .....(7.2)$$

Newton recognized that the higher the viscosity of a liquid, the greater is the shearing stress required to produce a certain rate of shear.

Hence, rate of shear should be directly proportional to shearing stress, (or)

$$\frac{F'}{A} \propto \frac{dv}{dr} \qquad \qquad .....(7.3)$$

$$\frac{F'}{A} = \eta \frac{dv}{dr} \qquad \qquad .....(7.4)$$

In eq. (7.4), η = Coefficient of viscosity or supply refereed as viscosity

Now eq. (7.4) can be rewritten as

$$F = \eta a \qquad \qquad .....(7.5)$$

$$\eta = \frac{F}{G} \qquad \qquad .....(7.6)$$

where, $F = F'/A$ and $G = dv/dr$

A rheogram (or) flow curve for a Newtonian system can be obtained by plotting 'F' versus 'a'.

It is shown in Fig. 7.2(a).

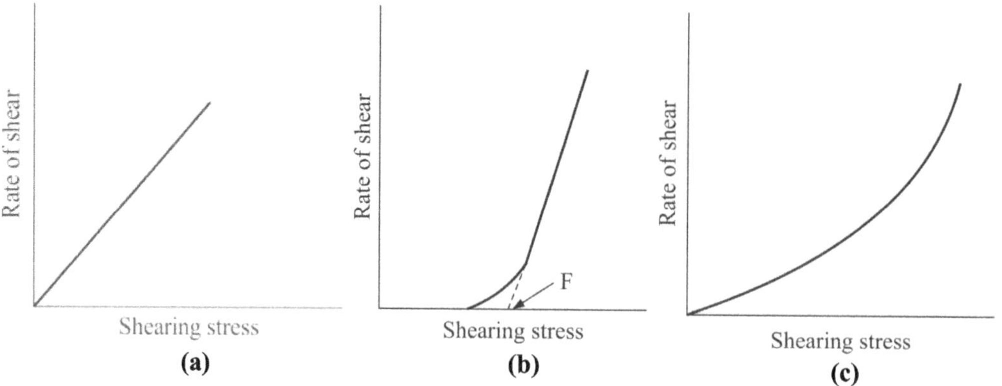

Fig.7.2 Representation flow curves for various materials.

As implied in eq. (7.6) a straight line is obtained which passes through the origin.

Rheograms are also known as consistency curves/flow curves and its slope – fluidity.

Advantage: Rheological properties of given material must completely described by its unique rheogram.

The viscosity of a fluid is the internal resistance or friction involved in the relative motion of one layer of molecules with respect to next.

The units of viscosity is the "poise", which can be defined in accordance with eq. (7.4) as the shearing force required to produce a velocity of 1 cm/sec between two parallel planes of liquid each 1 cm^2 in area and separated by a distance of 1 cm.

The CGS units for poise are dyne.sec/m^2 (or) g/cm.sec.

These can be obtained by dimensional analysis by rearranging eq. (7.4).

$$\eta = \frac{F'dr}{A\ dv} = \frac{dynes \times cm}{cm^2 \times cm/sec} = \frac{dyne.sec}{cm^2}$$

$$\frac{dyne.sec}{cm^2} = \frac{g \times cm/sec^2 \times sec}{cm^2} = \frac{g}{cm.sec}$$

The most convenient unit (or) most work is centipoise, cp.

    1 cp = 0.01 poise (or)

    1 poise = 100 cps.

The reciprocal of viscosity is known as fluidity and it is denoted by ϕ.

$$\phi = \frac{1}{\eta} \qquad\qquad .....(7.7)$$

Kinematic Viscosity is the absolute viscosity divided by the density of the liquid at a specific temperature.

$$\text{Kinematic Viscosity} = \frac{\eta}{\phi} \qquad \qquad .....(7.8)$$

Units are stoke(s) and centistoke (cs).

Relative Viscosity of a solution is the ratio of viscosity of a solution to the viscosity of its solvent

$$\eta_r = \frac{\eta}{\eta_o} \qquad \qquad .....(7.9)$$

η_r = Relative viscosity

η_o = Viscosity of solvent

Specific Viscosity can be written as

$$\eta_{sp} = \eta_r - 1 \qquad \qquad .....(7.10)$$

η_{sp} = Specific Viscosity

Table 7.1 Viscosity of some liquids commonly used in pharmacy are given in at 20 $^\circ$C.

Liquid	Viscosity (cp)
Castor oil	1000
Chloroform	0.563
Ethyl alcohol	1.19
Glycerine, 93%	400
Olive oil	100
Water	1.0019

7.2.2 Temperature Dependence and Theory of Viscosity

The viscosity of a liquid is decreases when temperature is raised (About 1-10% per $^\circ$C) where as fluidity increases.

The opposite effect may occur in certain cases.

E.g.: Aqueous solution of synthetic polymers like ethyl cellulose forms gel when temperature is increased.

Where as the viscosity of a gas increases with the temperature. In gases the molecules are in general so far and no appreciable intermolecular force exists and also kinetic movement of gas molecules are increased which causes an increase in viscosity.

The dependence of viscosity of liquid on temperature is expressed (for many substances) by Arrhenius equation of chemical kinetics.

$$\eta = A.e^{Ev\,RT} \qquad\qquad .....(7.11)$$

i.e.,
$$ln = \frac{Ev}{RT} + ln.A \qquad\qquad .....(7.12)$$

where, A = constant which depends on molecular weight and molar value as valve of liquid

E_v = Activation energy. Which is required to initiate flow feature molecules.

The energy required to remove a molecule from liquid (leaving a "hole" behind equal in size to that of molecule) is called energy of vaporisation.

The activation energy, E_v is found to be one-third of energy of vaporisation, because a molecule in flow can back, turn and maneuver in a space smaller than its actual size. Hence it can be concluded that free space required for flow is about 1/3rd the volume of molecule.

More energy is required to break the molecules associated through hydrogen bonds and to permit flow. This can be broken at higher temperature but E_v decreases.

Like fluidity, rate of diffusion increases exponentially with temperature.

7.3   Non–Newtonian Systems

Fluids that do not obey Newton's law are called Non-newtonian systems.

In these systems the value of 'η' (viscosity) varies with rate of shear.

Generally liquid & solid heterogeneous dispersions such as colloidal solution, emulsions liquid suspensions & ointments exhibit Non-newtonian behaviour.

When Non-newtonian materials are analyzed (in a rotational viscometer) and results are plotted. Various flow curves are obtained which represents their type of flow.

Mainly there are 3 classes of flow

1. Plastic
2. Pseudo plastic
3. Dilatant

7.3.1 Plastic Flow

There materials are known as Bingham bodies (in honor of 1st investigator to study plastic substances and also pioneer of modern Rheologys).

The flow curve/consistency curve is shown in Fig. 7.2(b). The curve does not pass through origin but if the straight part of the curve is extrapolated to the axis, it will intersect the shearing stress axis at one point known as yield value.

A Bingham body will flow only when shearing stress corresponding to yield value is exceeded. At below the yield value stress, it acts as elastic material.

Rheologists classifies the Brigham bodies into two types.

1. Solids – Substances exhibit a yield value

2. Liquids – Substances began to flow at smallest shearing stress and shows no yield value.

The slope of flow curve [in Fig. 7.2(b)] is termed as mobility (Analogous to fluidity). and its reciprocal is called plastic viscosity which is represented by 'U'.

$$U = \frac{F-f}{G} \qquad\qquad .....(7.13)$$

where, f = yield value/intercept on x-axis in dynes/cm^2

This type of flow is associated with presence of flocculated particles in concentrated suspensions, thereby which a continuous structure is exists throughout the system.

The yield value for these substances is due to contacts between adjacent particles (through van der Waals forces) and these must be broken down before flow can occur.

Therefore yield value is an indication of force of flocculation these are both are directly proportional. Frictional forces also contribute to yield value.

Once shearing stress (F – f) exceeds the yield value. Any further increasing of shear stress brings a directly proportional increase in G, (rate of shear).

At shear stress above yield value, plastic system resembles Newtonian system.

7.3.2 Pseudo Plastic Flow

These are also called shear thinning systems. It is exhibited by colloidal systems, especially polymer solutions and flocculated solid/liquid dispersions of Natural and synthetic gums (E.g., Tragacanth, sodium alginate etc.).

The type of rheogram obtained for these substances is shown in Fig. 7.2(c). The curve arises at the origin i.e., it has no yield value, because flow begins immediately on application of shearing stress. The slope of the curve gradually increases (until it reaches max. value)

Since the apparent viscosity at any shear rate is given by reciprocal of slope, the apparent viscosity decreases as shear rates increase (until a constant value is reached).

Since the curve is not linear, the viscosity of these materials cannot be expressed by any single value.

The curved rheogram for these materials results from a shearing action on long chain molecules of materials such as linear polymers. As shearing stress is increased, normally disarranged molecules begin to align their long axes in direction of flow, which reduces internal resistance of material. In addition, the solvent associated with the molecules may be released, resulting in effective lowering of the concentration and size of the dispersed molecules. This, too, will decrease apparent viscosity.

$$F^N = \eta'G \qquad\qquad\qquad .....(7.14)$$

The exponential formula has been found to represent the flow curve of some pseudo plastic materials.

Where in eq. (7.14), 'N' is indicative of Non-newtonian flow. The exponent N rises as flow becomes increasingly Non-newtonian.

When N = 1, the flow is Newtonian

η' = a viscosity coefficient.

Eq. (7.14) can be rearranged in logarithemic as

$$\text{Log } G = N \log F - \log \eta' \qquad\qquad .....(7.15)$$

This is an equation for a straight line. Many pseudo plastic systems fit this equation when log G is plotted as a function log F.

7.3.3   Dilatant Flow – Shear Thickening Systems

Certain suspensions with a high percentage of dispersed solids exhibit an increase in resistance to flow with increasing rates of shear. These systems actually increase in nature when sheared, hence these are termed as Dilatant, the flow is inverse of that possessed by pseudo plastic materials.

When stress is removed, a dilatant system returns to its original state of fluidity.

Eq. (7.14) can be used to describe dilatancy. 'N' is always less than 1 and decreases as degree of dilatancy increases.

As N = 1, the system becomes Newtonian in behaviour.

The suspensions containing a high concentration (about 50% or greater) of small, deflocculated particles possess dilatant flow properties.

Dilatant behaviour can be explained as follows.

At rest, particles are closely packed and having minimal inter particle volume. The amount of vehicle is sufficient to fill voids and permits particles to move relative to one another at low rates of shear can be pourable. As shear stress is increased, the bulk of system increases/dilates. Then particles take on an open form of packing as depicted in Fig. 7.3 which has large/increase in inter particular void volume. Since vehicle remains constant, it is insufficient to fill the increased voids increased resistance to flow is observed. Because, the particles are not completely wetted/lubricated by the vehicle. Suspension eventually becomes as a firm paste.

During processing of dilatant materials, appropriate precaution be used, otherwise these may solidify under high shear conditions and may damage high speed mixers, blenders or mills during processing.

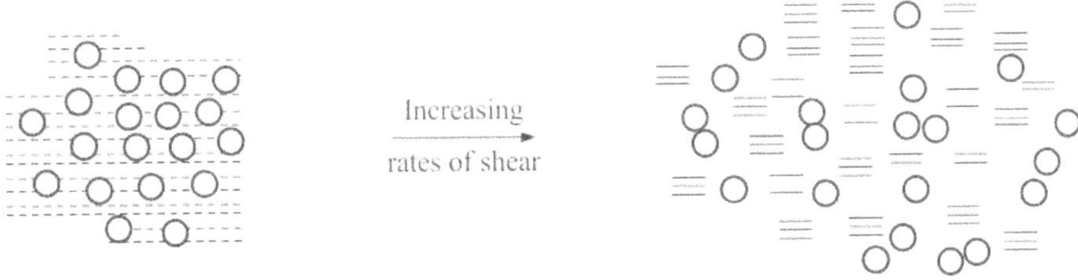

Fig. 7.3 Explanation of dilatant Flow behaviour.

7.4   Thixotropy

Thixotropy means "to change by touch".

For Newtonian systems, if a rheogram is plotted by increasing the rate of shear (as against shear stress) to desired maximum and then reduced, the down curve will superimpose on the curve.

But for Non-newtonian systems, the down curve will displaced to the left of the up curve (plastic and pseudo plastic). As shown in Fig. 7.4 which shows that the material has a lower consistency at any one rate of shear on down curve than it had on up curve. The structure do not reform immediately after stress is removed or reduced because of break down of structure. This is known as thixotrophy.

Thixotropy can be defined as an isothermal and comparatively slow recovery, on standing of a material, of a consistency lost through shearing.

It is applied only to shear-thinning system. A thixotropic system is a three dimensional network formed by (usually) asymmetric particles which are having numerous points of contact. This gives some degree of rigidity and at rest it resembles a get. When shear is applied, flow starts due to breakdown of points of contact and system undergoes get to solution formation (shear thinning) as particles get aligned. On removal of stress, the structure begins to reform, but not instantaneous. It is a progressive restoration of consistency as under random brownian movement, the asymmetric particles come into contact with one another.

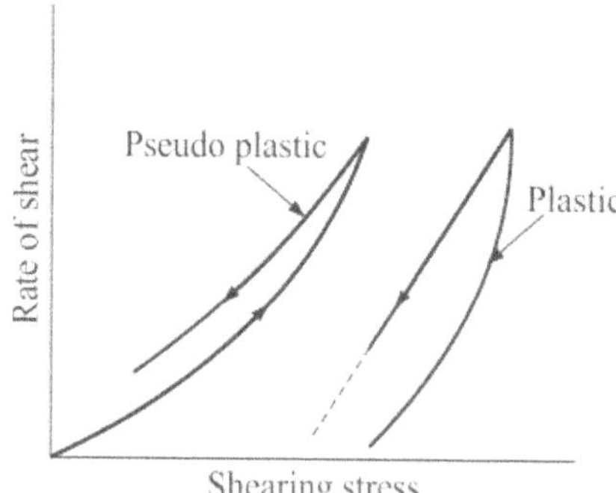

Fig. 7.4 Thixotropy in plastic and pseudoplastic flow systems.

Thixotropic rheograms obtained with thixotropic materials depend on

(i) Rate of shear

(ii) Length of time subjected to shear

7.4.1 Measurement of Thixotropy

An important/most characteristic of a thixotropic system is hysteresis loop which is formed by curve up down curves of rheogram and its area gives a measure of thixotropic breakdown.

To estimate the degree thixotropy for its Birgham bodies, two approaches are frequently used.

1. Determination of structural breakdown with time at a constant rate of shear.

   (a) In this method, shear rate is increased in a constant manner as shown in (Fig. 5). 'a' to 'b' and then decreased back to 'e' at the same rate.

   (b) A hysteresis loop "abe" is formed.

   (c) If the shear rate at point 'b' is held constant for 't', second (arbitrary), the shear stress and consistency decreases to an extent which depends on rate of shear, time of shear and degree of shear in sample.

   (d)   The decreasing in shear rate would result in hysteresis loop "abce".

   (e) If the rate of shear at point 'b' is held constant for 't_2' seconds, the loop abcde will be observed.

A rheogram of a thixotropic material will depend on rheologic history of sample and the method used to obtain the rheogram.

The thixotropic coefficient B, the rate of breakdown with time of constant shear rate is calculated from

$$B = \frac{U_1 - U_2}{ln\frac{t_2}{t_1}} \qquad\qquad .....(7.16)$$

where, U_1 and U_2 are plastic viscosities of 2 down curves, after shearing at a constant rate for t_1 and t_2 seconds respectively.

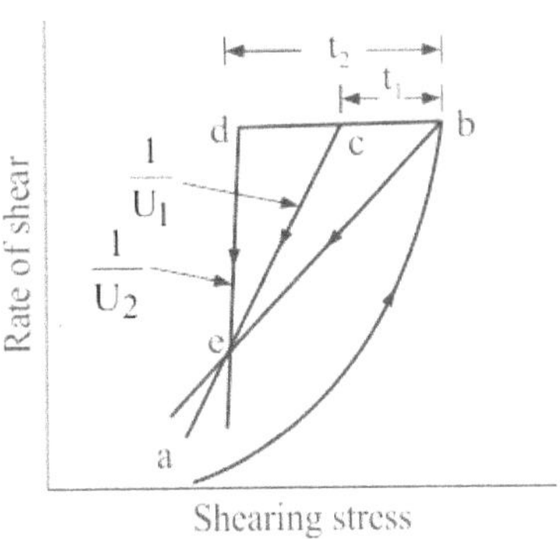

Fig. 7.5 Structural breakdown with time of a plastic system possessing thixotropy when subjected to a constant rate of shear for t_1 and t_2 seconds.

2. Determination of structural breakdown due to increasing shear rate (or) fall in shear with time at rates of shear

   (a) The principle involved shown in Fig.7.6.

   (b) By applying 2 different maximum rates of shear v_1 and v_2 we can obtain 2 hysteresis loops.

   (c) The loss in shearing, shear per unit increase in shear rate is called thirotrophic coefficient M, which is obtained from

$$M = \frac{U_1 - U_2}{ln\left(\frac{V_2}{V_1}\right)} \qquad\qquad .....(7.17)$$

where, M = thirotropic coefficient in dynes sec/m^2

U_1 and U_2 = plastic viscosities for 2 down curves having maximum shears rate of v_1 and v_2 respectively.

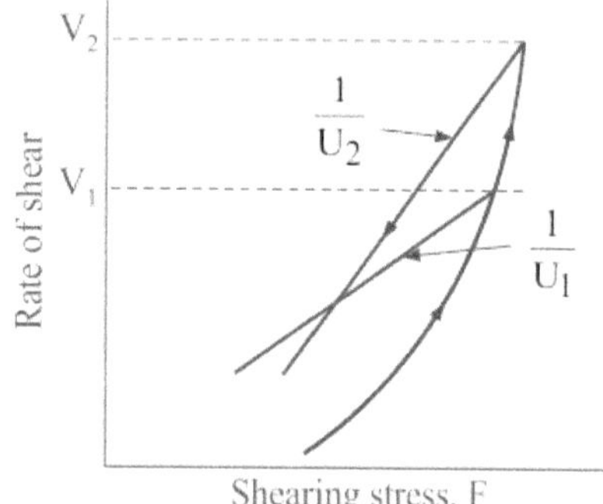

Fig. 7.6 Structural breakdown of a plastic system possessing thixotropy when subjected to increasing shear rates.

Disadvantages

1. Time consuming
2. 'M' will depend on v_1 and v_2 (arbitrarily chosen) which will affect the down curves and hence the values of 'U' that are calculated.

7.4.2 Bulges and Spurs

The dispersions which are employed in pharmacy may yield complex hysteresis loops in their rheograms. These are may be a "bulge" or "spur".

As shown in Fig. 7.7 for aqeous bentonite gel, (10 – 15% by wt) produces a hysteresis loop which has bulge in up curve, due to formation of "have-of-clouds" structure by crystalline plates of bentonite and this structure causes swelling of bentonite magmas.

As shown in Fig.7.8. for more lightly structured systems, bulged curve develop into a spur like protrusion.

E.g.: Procaine penicillin (3 ml injection).

The structures demonstrates a spur value, which represents a sharp point of structural breakdown at low shear rate.

The spur value, is obtained by using an instrument in which rate of shear can be slowly and uniformly increased, preferably automatically and shear stress read out or plotted on an x-y recorder, as a function of shear rate.

7.4.3 Negative Thixotropy/Anti Thixotropy

It represents an increasing in consistency on down curve rather than decreasing consistency, as in previous cases, on the materials, system, with increase in shear rate. The thickness and resistance to flow increases.

It is observed in Magnesia magma (but not in pharmaceutical system).

The anti-thixotropic character of magnesia magma is demonstrated in Fig. 7.9.

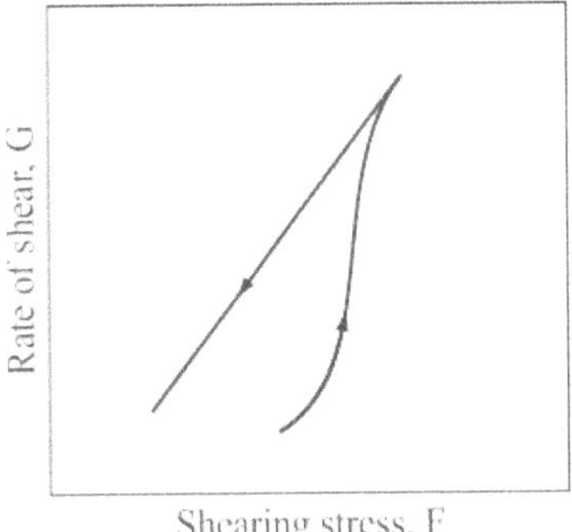

Fig. 7.7 Rheogram of thixotropic material showing a bulge in the hysteresis loop.

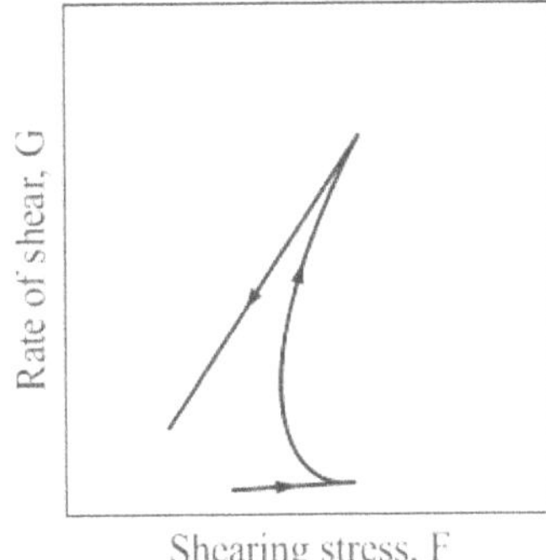

Fig. 7.8 Rheogram of thixotropic material showing a spur value r in the hysteresis loop.

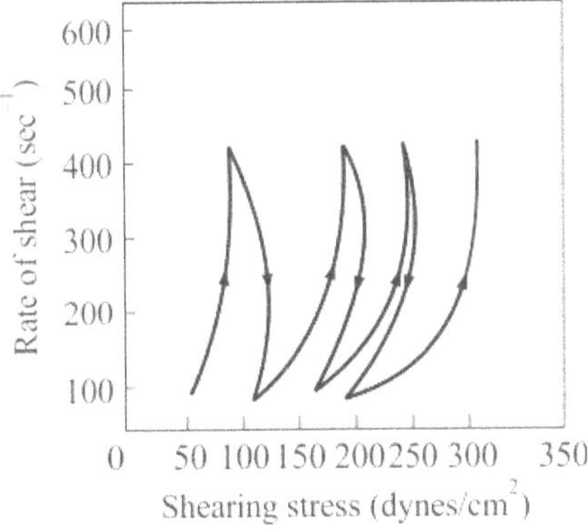

Fig. 7.9 Rheogram of Magnesia magma showing antithixotropic behaviour. The material is sheared at repeated increasing and then decreasing rates of shear at stage D, further cycling no longer increased the consistency, and the upcurves and downcurves coincided.

When it was sheared at alternative rates, the magma continuously thickened, but at a decreasing rate and finally reached an equilibrium state in which further increasing material decreasing shear rates no longer increased the consistency of material.

At equilibrium state, it was found to be like and readily pourable, on standing it returned to its solution like properties.

It is different from

1. Dilatancy and

2. Rheopexy

Dilatant system	Anti Thixotropic system
(a) Contains greater than 50% by volume of solid phase	(a) Contains low solid content, about 1-10%
(b) Solids are in deflocculated state	(b) Solids are in flocculated state

Rheopexy	Anti-thixotropy
Gel is equilibrium state	Solution is equilibrium state

Rheopexy is a phenomenon in which a solid forms a gel more readily when taken gently (or) otherwise sheared, than when allowed to form the gel while the material is kept at rest.

Note: The assessment of thixotropic products requires rotational viscometry in order to plot up and down curves.

Applications

1. It is particularly useful in formulation of suspension & emulsion.

    A thixotropic agent such as Bentonite, Magnesium magma, silicon dioxide etc. Carter a high apparent viscosity/a yield value which will retard sedimentation or creaming which are main problems in formulation of suspensions and emulsions.

    At greater stresses than yield value, the formulation can be pourable and at rest, the viscosity slowly increases and yield value is restored because of regain of 3-dimensional structure.

2. It is also helpful/desirable property with lotions, creams, ointments (easily spreadable).

3. It is an important desirable property in formulation of parenteral suspensions which are meant for intramuscular depot therapy.

    E.g.: Procaine penicillin G parenteral suspension contains 40-70% w/v has a high inherent thixotropy.

    When it passes through the hypodermic needle, breakdown of structure occurs and the consistency was recovered as rheological structure reformed. Which leads to formation of depot of drug at I.M injection site and drug was slowly released and available for long time.

7.5   Determination of Rheological Properties

7.5.1   Choice of Viscometer

The determination and evaluation of rheological properties of any material depends on choosing the correct instrument method.

For Newtonian systems, "Single-point" instruments are used. Which operate at single shear rate, because in these systems, rate of shear is directly proportional to shearing stress.

The single point obtained by these instruments can extrapolate to origin and a complete rheogram can be obtained.

For Non-newtonian systems, these are unsuitable, because they are unable to describe the changes which are occurring in the systems during agitating, paining etc.

For Non-newtonian materials/systems/systems, only "multi-point" instruments are used which has variable shear rate controls.

All viscometers can be used to determine the viscosities of Newtonian systems.

Single-point Instrument- E.g.: Capillary and falling sphere viscometer – only for Newtonian liquids.

Multi-point Instrument- E.g.: Cup and bob and

Cone and plate – for both Newtonian and Non-Newtonian system.

7.5.2   Types of Rheological Instruments

1. Capillary or Tube Viscometer

    E.g.: Ostwald Viscometer

2. Couette or Rotational Viscometer

    E.g.: Brookfield Viscometer

3. Cone and Plate Viscometers

    E.g.: Ferranti-Shirley Viscometer

4. Density-Dependent Viscometer

    E.g.: Falling Sphere Viscometer

    Hoeppler Viscometer

5. Penetrometers - Measure the hardness/clustery of relatively rigid semi-solids

    E.g.: Cone and Needle forms are commonly used

7.5.3 Principle Methods for Measuring Viscosity

There are 3 methods

1. Based on rate of flow of a liquid through an orifice or a duct.

    E.g.: Capillary viscometer

2. Based on the resistance of a rotating element in contact with or immersed in the liquid.

    E.g.: Concentric cylinder viscometer

3. Based on the velocity of an object rolling or falling through the liquid under the effect of gravity.

    E.g.: Rolling/falling sphere viscometer

In this chapter, we are discussing only some important viscometers which are generally used.

7.5.4 Capillary Viscometer/Ostwald's Viscometer

It is used to determine the viscosities of Newtonian fluids.

Principle: The rate of flow of fluid through the capillary is measured under the influence of gravity (or) an externally applied pressure.

In this method, viscosity can be determined by measuring the time required for the liquid to pass between two marks as it flows by gravity through a vertical capillary tube known as ostwald viscometer, which is shown in Fig. 7.10. The time of flow of liquid under test is compared with the time required for a liquid known viscosity (usually water) to pass between two marks.

The absolute viscosity of unknown liquid η_1, is determined by

$$\frac{\eta_1}{\eta_2} = \frac{\rho_1 t_1}{\rho_2 t_2} \qquad\qquad .....(7.18)$$

where, η_1 and η_2 are viscosities of unknown and standard liquids respectively.

ρ_1 and ρ_2 - Respective densities of liquids

t_1 and t_2 - Respective flow times in sec.

The ratio $\eta_1/\eta_2 = \eta_{rel}$ which is known as relative viscosity

The Eq. (7.18) is based on Poiseuille's law for a liquid flowing through a capillary tube.

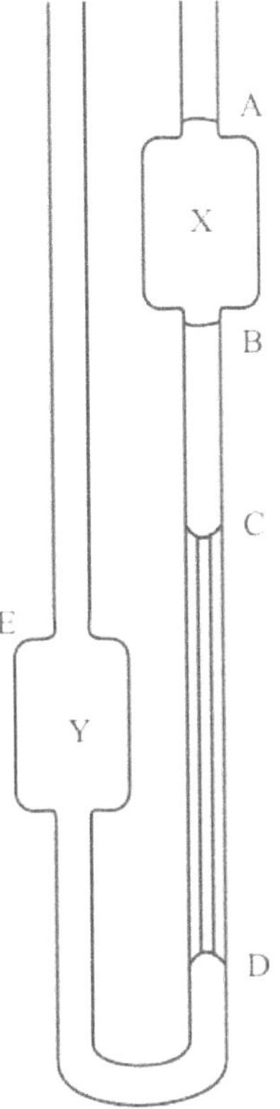

Fig. 7.10 Ostwald viscometer.

$$\eta = \frac{\pi r^4 t\, \Delta P}{8 l V} \qquad\qquad\qquad \text{.....(7.19)}$$

where r = radius of inside of capillary

t = time of flow

ΔP = pressure head (m dyne/cm^2) under which liquid flows

l = length of capillary tube

V = volume of liquid flowing

Since, the length, volume and radius of a given capillary viscometer are invariants, they are combined into a constant, K.

Eq. (7.19) can be written as

$$\eta = k t\, \Delta P \qquad\qquad\qquad \text{.....(7.20)}$$

The pressure head ΔP depends on

h = height of liquid levels in two arms

ρ = density of liquid

δ = acceleration due to gravity

If the liquids levels in the capillary are kept constant, (according of gravity is constant).

Eq. (7.20) becomes as

$$\eta = k't\rho \qquad\qquad .....(7.21)$$

For unknown and standard liquids it becomes

$$\eta_1 = k'\, t_1\, \rho_1 \qquad\qquad .....(7.22)$$

$$\eta_2 = k'\, t_2\, \rho_2 \qquad\qquad .....(7.23)$$

During comparison of unknown and standard liquids, the division of Eq. (7.22) by Eq. (7.22), (7.23) gives Eq. (7.18).

Procedure/Method: Ostwald's viscometer consists of U-tube bearing two bulbs x and y and in one arm. It is written as "fine capillary CD" of suitable bore. It is placed vertically in thermostatically controlled bath. The liquid, viscosity to be determined, is poured into bulb 'y' to reach mark. The liquid is sucked up to a point A; the time (t_1) for liquid to fall from A to B is measured in sec (using stop watch). The density of liquid (ρ_1) is also determined. It is repeated for often solvents.

Then ρ_2 and t_2 are determined. Then viscosity can be determined from Eq. (7.18).

Disadvantages

1. Determination of viscosity of highly viscous liquids in a standard ostwald's will not give accurate a viscosity.

2. Care should be taken not to introduce air bubbles.

This problem can be avoided by using suspended level viscometer which is shown in Fig. 7.11. In this, an additional side arm 'c' ensure the entry of capillary is at atmosphere pressure, so that the total amount of liquid in viscosity does not require to be fixed. It can be used for determining the amount of methyl cellulose solution.

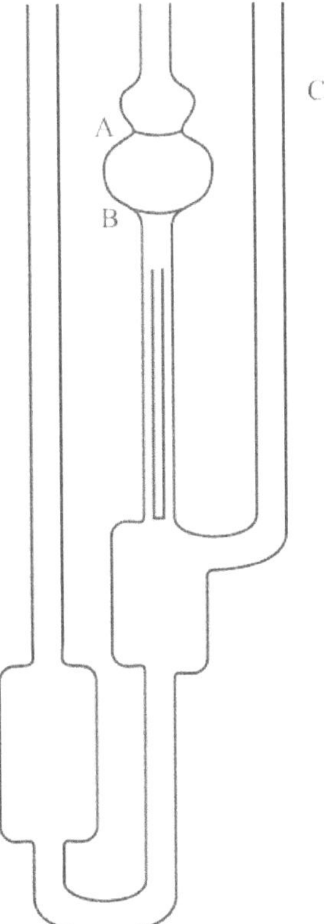

Fig. 7.11 Suspended level viscometer.

7.5.5 Falling Sphere Viscometer

For Newtonian liquids Hoeppler falling sphere viscometer is used. As shown in Fig. 7.12 a glass or steel ball rolls down in vertical glass tube containing the test liquid at a known constant temperature.

Principle: The rate at which a ball of a particular density and diameter falls is an inverse function of viscosity of sample.

The sample and ball are placed in inner a glass tube which is surrounded by constant-temp. Jacked and teen the tube and jacket are inverted which places the ball at top of inner glass tube.

The time for ball to fall between two marks is accurately measured and repeated for several times.

The viscosity of Newtonian liquids can be determined from

$$\eta = t\,(s_b - s_f)\,B \qquad . \qquad\qquad\qquad .....(7.24)$$

where, t = time interval in sec for ball to fall between two marks

s_b = specific gravity of ball

s_f = specific gravity of fluid

B = a constant for a particular ball and supplied by manufactures

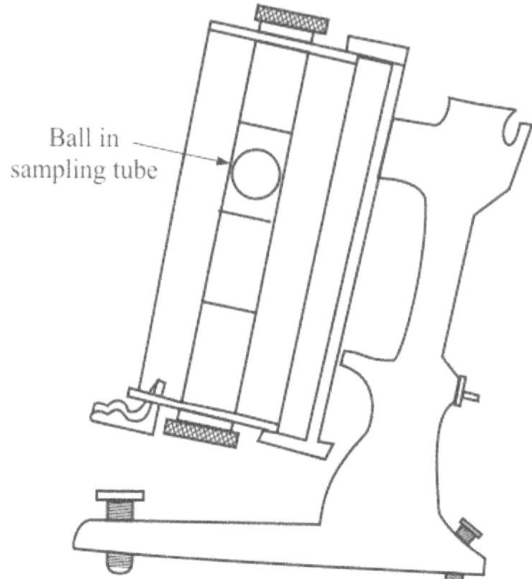

Fig. 7.12 Hoeppler falling ball viscometer.

Advantages

1. This instrument can be used for viscosities over the range of 0.5 - 2,00,000 poise as variety of glass and steel balls of difference diameters are available.

   For best results, a ball should be used such that 't' is not less than 30 sec.

2. The method is capable of high precision provided that adequate temperature control is maintained.

7.5.6 Rotational Viscometers

These instruments relay on the viscous drug exerted on a body when it is rotated in the fluid to determine its viscosity.

Major Advantage: Wide range of shear rate can be achieved and the flow curve of a material may be obtained directly.

Couette type and cone and plate are generally preferred viscometers.

7.5.7 Cop and Bob Viscometer

In these viscometers the sample is sheared in the space between outer wall of a bob and inner wall of a cup into which bob fits.

Based on rotation of cup/bob, these are divided into 2 types.

1. **Couette type of viscometer:** In this, cup is rotated, the viscous drag on the bob is due to sample canes it to turn. The resultant torque is proportional to viscosity of sample.

   E.g.: MacMicheal viscometer

2. **Searle type of viscometer:** Here the cup is stationary and bob is rotated. The viscous drag of system is measured by spring/sensor introduce to the bob.

   E.g.: Rotovisco Viscometer

A popular instrument based on Searle principle is the shower instrument. The principle involved is shown in Fig. 7.13. The modification of that viscometer is described by Fischer and it is shown in Fig. 7.14.

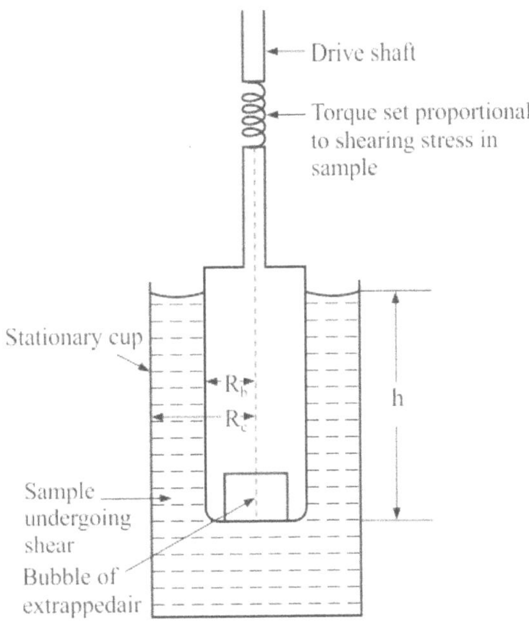

Fig. 7.13 Principle of rotational cup and bob viscometer.

The test system is placed in the space between the cup and bob and allowed to reach temperature equilibrium. The time required for the bob to make 100 revolutions is recorded by placing the weight on hanger. The data obtained is converted into rpm. The weight is increased and whole procedure is repeated.

A Rheogram can be constructed by plotting rpm verses weight added.

By use of appropriate constants, rpm values are converted to actual shear rates in $\sec^{-1}$ and weights into units of shear stress namely, dynes/cm^2.

For a rotational viscometer, Eq. (7.4) becomes as

$$\Omega = \frac{1}{\eta} \frac{T}{4\pi h}\left(\frac{1}{R_b^2} - \frac{1}{R_c^2}\right)$$

.....(7.25)

where, Ω = angular velocities in radians/sec

T = torque in dynes cm.

h = the depth to which bob is immersed in liquid

R_b and R_c = radius of bob and cup respectively.

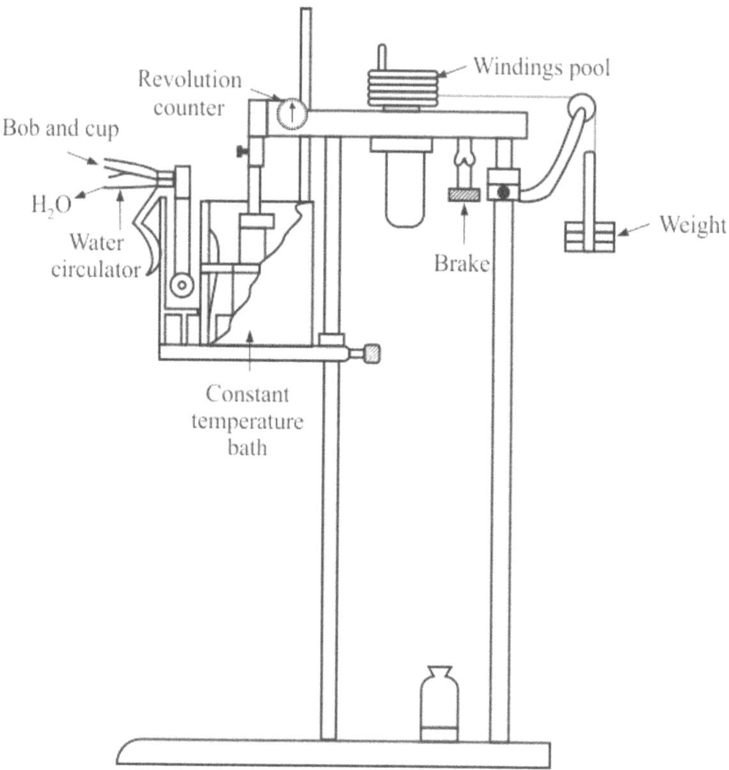

Fig. 7.14 Stormer viscometer the falling weights cause the bob to rotate in the stationary cup. The velocity of bob is obtained by means of a stop watch and revolution centre.

Note: The stormer instrument should not be used with systems having a viscosity below 20 cp.

The viscous drag of the sample on the bare of the bob is not taken into account (A pocket of air is entrapped between sample and bare of bob renders the contribution from bare of bob negligible).

By combining all the constants eq. (7.25) can be written as

$$\eta = k_v \frac{T}{\Omega} \qquad\qquad .....(7.26)$$

k_v = can be determined by analysing an oil of known viscosity in the instrument

Employing stormer instrument, the eq for plastic viscosity is

$$U = k_v \frac{w - w_f}{v} \qquad\qquad .....(7.27)$$

where,   U = plastic viscosity in poises

w_f = yield value in gm

The yield value of plastic system is obtained by

$$F = k_f \times w_f \qquad\qquad .....(7.28)$$

where, k_f is equal to

$$k_f = k_v \times \frac{2\pi}{60} \times \frac{1}{2.303 \, \log\left(R_c/R_b\right)} \qquad\qquad .....(7.29)$$

Applications

1. Used in quality control laboratories.
2. A number of spinders/bobs of various geometries including cylinder, t-bonds etc. are available which provides data for both Newtonian and Non-newtonian liquids.
3. It also provides empirical viscosity measurements on paster and other semi-solid materials.

7.5.8 Cone and Plate Viscometer

E.g.: Ferranti-shirley viscometer

The sample is placed at centre of plate which is then moved into position under the cone, as shown in Fig.7.15. The measuring unit of apparatus is shown Fig. 7.16.

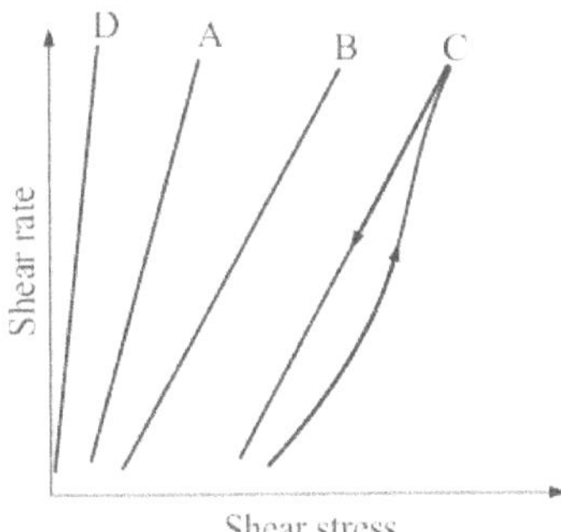

Fig. 7.15 Flow curves of kaolin suspension in water A – 20% w/v, B – 30% w/v, C – 40% w/v, D – 40% w/v 10% sodium citrate.

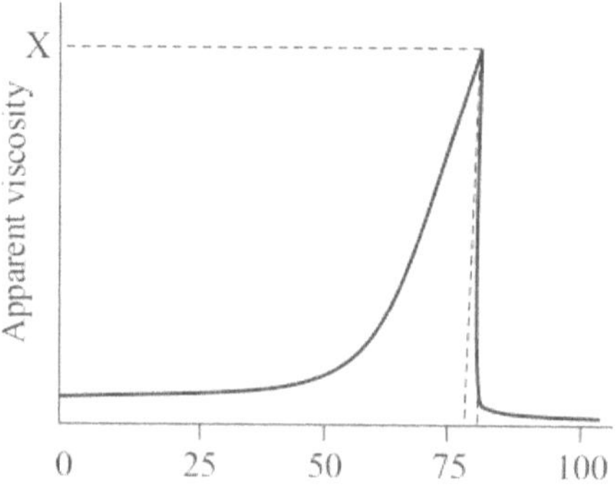

Fig. 7.16 Variation of apparent viscosity with volume concentration (percent) of water in a water-in-oil emulsions maximum viscosity at x-inversion beyond this point.

The sample is sheared in narrow gap between plate (stationary) and cone, which is driven by various speed motor. The shear rate in rpm is increased and decreased by a selector dial and shearing stress (torque) produced on cone is read on the indicator scale.

A plot of shear rate (rpm) and shearing stress can be constructed.

The viscosity of Newtonian liquid can be measured in poise, by below equation

$$\eta = C\frac{T}{V} \qquad \qquad .....(7.30)$$

where, C = instrumental constant

     T = Torque reading

     V = Speed of cone in rpm

For a material shows plastic flow, plastic viscosity is given by

$$U = C\frac{T - T_f}{V} \qquad \qquad .....(7.31)$$

And yield value, is given by

$$f = C_f \times T_f \qquad \qquad .....(7.32)$$

T_f = Torque at shearing stress axis (extrapolated from linear portion of curve)

C_f = Instrument constant

As shown in Fig.7.15. (principle), that rate of shear, a, at any dielectric is directly proportional to ratio of linear velocity, Ωr, to the gap width, d. Thus

$$G = \frac{\Omega r}{d} \; \frac{cm/sec}{cm} \qquad \qquad .....(7.33)$$

The ratio r/d is proportional to angle between cone and plate, ψ , in radians

Then $$G = \frac{\Omega}{\psi} \ \sec^{-1} \qquad\qquad .....(7.34)$$

Ω = rotation (rad/sec)

ψ = cone angle (rad)

It is independent of radius of cone and cone angle generally ranges from $0.3 - 4°$.

The instrument can be modified to allow the simultaneous recording of shear rate and stress along shearing constant acceleration of cone, so that flow curves can be obtained automatically on an x-y recorder.

The control unit permits different rates of acceleration and deceleration of cone, so that rheological properties of fluids of thixotropic materials can be studied.

Automatic recording of flow curves is particularly useful when rapid changes of viscosity occurs on shearing, as there may be missed when operates the instrument manually.

Advantages

1. Uniform rate of shear across sample, so chance of plus flow is avoided.
2. Sample requires only 0.1-0.2 ml.

   (whereas cup and bob viscosities require 20-50 ml)
3. Good temperature control
4. Easy to clean
5. Automatic recording allows flow curves to be obtained quickly and under standardized conditions.

Disadvantages

1. Unsuitable for coarse suspensions and emulsions because of narrow clearance between cone and plate.
2. Suspension of particles of size not greater than 30 μm can be sheared in standard cone $(0.3°)$.

Applications

1. Used for measuring rheological properties of ointment bases.
2. Used for both Newtonian and Non-Newtonian fluids.

In case of Newtonian fluids, a caution should be taken. If rapid acceleration – deceleration is applied to liquids, may produce erroneous results and inaccurate hysteresis loops may be obtained.

7.5.9 Visco Elastic Materials

The materials which exhibit both viscous properties of liquids and elastic properties of solids

E.g.: Creams, lotions, ointments, suppositories, suspending agents, biological materials such as blood, sputum and chemical fluids etc.

For evaluating visco elastic materials creep and oscillatory method are useful.

Applications to Pharmacy

1. The rheological behaviour of poloxamer vehicles was studied as a function of concentration over a temperature range of 5 °C-35 °C using cone and plate viscometer.
2. Using computer-controlled couette viscometer, we can study rheological properties of substances like sodium hyaluronate solution.
3. By using a rotational viscometer, the rheological properties of triglyceride suppository base at various temperatures can be studied.
4. By use of Brookfield digital viscometer curve, rheological properties of mineral-oil-water emulsions stabilized with triethanolamine stearate, was studied (as function of temperature).
5. The rheological properties of microcrystalline cellulose (An ingredient which facilitates granulation) can be studied with the help of mixer torque rheometer
6. In formulation and analysis of various products like suppaiture, embious etc.

   in addition to the applications given under individual viscometer.

7.5.10 Pharmaceutical Areas in which Rheology is significant

1. Fluids

   (a) Mixing

   (b) Particle size reduction of disperse systems with shear

   (c) Fluid transfer, including pumping and flow through pipes

2. Quasi solids

   (a) Spreading and adherence on the skin

3. Solids

   (a) Flow of powders from hopper and into die cavities in tabletting into capsules drug encapsulation.

   (b) Packagability of powdered/granular solid.

4. Processing

   (a) Processing efficiency

   (b) Production capacity of equipment

7.6   Rheology of Suspensions

The viscosity of the liquid increases by the addition of a disperse phase, due to disturbance of stream lines of liquid around the particle.

Einstein developed a theoretical expression relating the viscosity of suspension (η), to the volume fraction (ϕ) of particles

$$\eta = \eta_0 \,(1 + 2.5\phi) \qquad\qquad .....(7.35)$$

where, η_0 = viscosity of the vehicle

η = viscosity of disperse system i.e., suspension

The eq. (7.35) is only applicable to very dilute suspensions of rigid spherical particles. For suspensions containing higher concentrations,

$$\eta = \eta_0 \,(1 + 2.5\,\phi + k_1\phi^2 + k_2\phi^3 ....)$$

have been developed,

where, k_1 and k_2 are the constant for the system.

The particle shape, particle size distribution and degree of flocculation of the particles play an important role in determining the flow properties of suspensions (particularly if the concentration of disperse phase is high).

E.g.: If the particles are more uniform, the viscosity of suspensions is higher, for a given concentration of solid.

The properties of suspensions must be adjusted so that:

1. The product must be easily administered

    E.g.: It must be easily poured from a bottle (or) forced through a syringe needle.
2. Sedimentation is either prevented or retarded. If sedimentation occur, redispersion is easy.
3. The product has an elegance appearance.

The variation of flow properties of suspensions such as kaolin and barium sulphate in water as the concentration is increased.

By the addition of sodium citrate, the viscosity is reduced and is shown in curve D.

The rheological properties of suspensions as discussed previously changes/affected by degree of flocculation, because the amount of free continuous phase is reduced, as it becomes entrapped in the diffuse floccules.

Flocculated suspensions tend to exhibit plastic or pseudoplastic behaviour, while deflocculated suspensions tend to be dilatants i.e., that the apparent viscosity of flocculated suspensions is high when the applied shearing stress is low and it decreases as applied stress increases. If a system exhibits plastic flow, then it behaves like a solid upto yield value and no flow is occurs until this value is exceeded. The apparent viscosity of deflocculated suspensions is low at low shearing stress and increases as applied stress increases.

Deflocculated suspensions are easy to pour, where as flocculated ones are not, since shearing stress involved in pouring are relatively low. Dilatant systems may sieze up the mill during operation due to high speed which causes increases in viscosity.

7.6.1 Deflocculated Particles in Newtonian Vehicles

When these systems sediment, a compact cake is produced, which causes problem to redisperse. The rate of sedimentation can be reduced by increasing the viscosity of the continuous medium.

However, it presents/causes the problem during pouring of suspension from bottle and also, if sedimentation occurs, it offers much more problem (or) resistance to redisperse the cake.

7.6.2 Deflocculated Particles in Non-Newtonian Particles

Only pseudoplastic or plastic dispersions media can be used in the formulation of suspensions and both will retard the sedimentation of small particles, as their apparent viscosities will be higher under the small stress associated with sedimentation. The hydrocolloids used as suspending agents such as Acacia, Tragacanth, Gelatin etc. will impart Non-Newtonian properties to suspensions. The 3 dimensional gel network traps deflocculated particles at rest and their sedimentation is retarded and may be completely prevented.

7.6.3 Flocculated Particles in Newtonian Vehicles

The flocculated particles will sediment, but aggregates are diffuse, a large volume of sediment is produced and which is easier to disperse. But the problem is it causes inelegance to the suspension because the sediment does not fill whole of the fluid volume.

7.6.4 Flocculated Particles in Non-Newtonian Vehicles

This type of system allows the advantages to previous 2 methods to be utilised. Variations in the properties of material to be suspended are less likely to influence the performance of a product made on a large scale, and less difference will be observed between batches of product made from the same flow sheet.

7.7   Rheology of Emulsions

When droplets of one liquid are emulsified in an immiscible liquid, the viscosity of continuous phase is increases. Einstein equation which is given in previous section is also applicable to emulsions.

With the variation of volume concentration of disperse phase, the apparent viscosity changes [sometimes it may leads to phase inversion]. It is shown that in Fig. 7.1. The maximum (theoretical) volume of internal phase is 74% v/v, but droplets are not uniform, so smaller drops can pack between the larger ones. The viscosity of internal phase has no effect on the (little effect sometimes) emulsion.

Except very dilute emulsions, others are non-newtonian and their apparent viscosity decreases with increase in rate of shear.

The fluid emulsions are usually pseudoplastic and those approading a semi-solid nature behave plastically and exhibit marked yield value. The semi-solid creams are usually visco elastic. The emulsifying agent can be used to carter viscoelastic properties on a topical cream merely by varying the ratio of surface-active agent to long-chain alcohol.

Pharmaceutical emulsions often exhibit some degree of thixotropy.

The important factors influencing viscosity of emulsions are:

1. Internal phase

    (a) viscosity; deformation of globules in shear

    (b) globules size and size distribution, technique used to prepare emulsion, globule behaviour in shear, globule interaction

2. Continuous phase

    (a) Viscosity,

    (b) Chemical constitution, polarity, pH; potential energy of interaction between globules

    (c) Electrolyte concentration of polar medium

3. Emulsifying agent

    (a) Chemical constitution

    (b) Concentration and solubility in internal and external phases; emulsion type, emulsion inversion, solubilisation of liquid phases in micelles

    (c) Thickness of film adsorbed around globules

    (d) Electroviscous effect

4. Additional effect

    (a) Pigments, hydrocolloids, hydrous oxides

    (b) Effect on rheological properties of liquid phases and interfacial boundary region

Auxan showed that increasing quantities of cetyl alcohol produced an increase in both yield value and plastic viscosity of emulsions.

Talman, Davies and Rowan studied the rheology of similar emulsions and suggested that the large increase in viscosity as the cetostearyl alcohol was increased, was due to formation of gel in the aqueous phase due to the interaction of alcohol with sodium lauryl sulphate. Get formation would play a dominant role in the viscosity of emulsions containing emulsifying waxes.

Rheology of semi-solids

A semi-solid is having both solid and liquid characters.

The flow of a Newtonian fluid is given by

$$\eta = F/G \qquad\qquad .....(7.36)$$

Relating shear stress F and shear rate 'G'.

A solid material is characterised by elasticity rather than flow and its behaviour is expressed as the equation for spring is

$$E = F/\gamma \qquad\qquad .....(7.37)$$

where, E = Elastic modulus dyne/cm^2

F = Stress dyne/cm^2

γ = Strain

A viscous fluid may be given as movement of a piston in a cylinder (dashpot) (a) filled with a liquid,

E.g.: For dashpot is automobile shock absorber.

The behaviour of a semi solid, a visco elastic body may be described by combination of dash pot and spring (c):

The mechanical model of visco elastic body, a combination of dashpot and spring in series is Maxwell unit/element. The parallel arrangement of dashpot and spring is voigt elements.

When a constant stress is applied on Maxwell unit, there is a strain of material causing displacement of spring. The applied stress also produces a movement of the piston in the dashpot, due to viscous flow. Removal of stress leads to complete recovery of spring, but no recovery in viscous flow.

In the voigt, the drag of viscous fluid in the dashpot influences the extension and compression of spring and the strain is expressed as deformation (J) of the text material and it is the strain per unit stress. The deformation of visco elastic material by voigt model as a function of time t, is given by

$$J = J_\infty \left(1 - e^{-t/\tau}\right) \qquad\qquad .....(7.38)$$

In which J_∞ = deformation at infinite time

τ = viscosity per unit modulus $\left(\eta/E\right)$

which is called as retardation time.

Deformations are compliance (J) as the function of time is measured with creep viscometer and when compliance and time are plotted creep curve is obtained. Creep curve consists of three parts sharply raising portion (AB) represents the elastic movement of the spring.

Curved position (BC) represents viscometer region which is the action of two voigt units.

A linear position (CD) represents the movement of the piston is the dashpot at the bottom of Maxwell-Voigt Model representing viscous flow.

CHAPTER 8

DISPERSED SYSTEMS

8.1 Suspensions

A suspension is a particular class or type of dispersion or dispersed system in which the internal or suspended phase is dispersed uniformly by mechanical agitation throughout the external phase (called the suspending medium or vehicle).

The internal phase has specific size range for the correct distribution of solid particles. In a colloidal dispersion of suspension, the solids are less than about 1 μm in size. In a coarse suspension, they are larger than about 1 μm. The practical upper limit for individual suspending particle is 50-75 μm in coarse dispersions.

Oral antibiotic syrups are the examples of oral suspensions which has 125-500 mg per 5 ml of solid material. When formulated as pediatric drops the concentration of suspended material is correspondingly increased. Antacid and radioopaque suspension generally contain high concentration of dispersed solids. In external preparation it may increase to 20% or more. Parenteral suspensions contain 0.5-30% of solid particles. Viscosity and particle size are significant factors because they affect the ease of injection and the availability of the drug in depot therapy.

8.2 Interfacial Properties of Suspended Particles

Knowledge of thermodynamic requirements is needed for the successful stabilization of suspended particles.

Work must be done to reduce a solid to small particles and disperse them in a continuous medium. The large surface area of the particles that results from the comminution is associated with surface free energy that makes the system "thermodynamically unstable", by which particles are highly energetic and tend to regroup to lessen the surface area and reduce surface free energy. The particles therefore tend to flocculate, that is, to form, fluffy agglomerates that are held together by weak van der Waals forces. In a compacted cake particles may adhere by stronger forces to form what are termed aggregates. Caking occurs by growth and fusing of crystals in

152

An increase in the work w, or surface free energy, ΔG, brought about by dividing the solid into smaller particles and consequently increasing the total surface area ΔA is given by

$$\Delta G = r_{SL} \cdot \Delta A \qquad\qquad .....(8.1)$$

where, r_{SL} = interfacial tension between the liquid medium and the solid particles.

To approach a stable system, the system tends to reduce the surface free energy, equilibrium is reached when $\Delta G = 0$. This condition can be accomplished, as seen from equation (8.1) by reducing interfacial tension.

The interfacial tension can be reduced by addition of surface active agents but cannot be made to zero. A suspension of insoluble particles, then usually possesses a finite positive interfacial tension, and the particles tend to flocculate.

The potential energy of two particles are plotted in Fig. 8.1(a) as a function of the distance of separation, shown are the curves depicting the energy of attraction, the energy of repulsion and the net energy of attraction, the energy of repulsion and the net energy which has a peak and two minima. When the repulsion energy is high, the potential barrier is also high and the collision of the particles is apposed, Fig. 8.1(b) shows variation is net potential of interactions. When particles are flocculated, the energy barrier is still too large to be surmounted, and so approaching particle resides in second energy minima which is at a distance of separation of perhaps 1000-2000 A°. This distance is sufficient for formation of loosely formed flocs. These concepts evolve from DLVO theory.

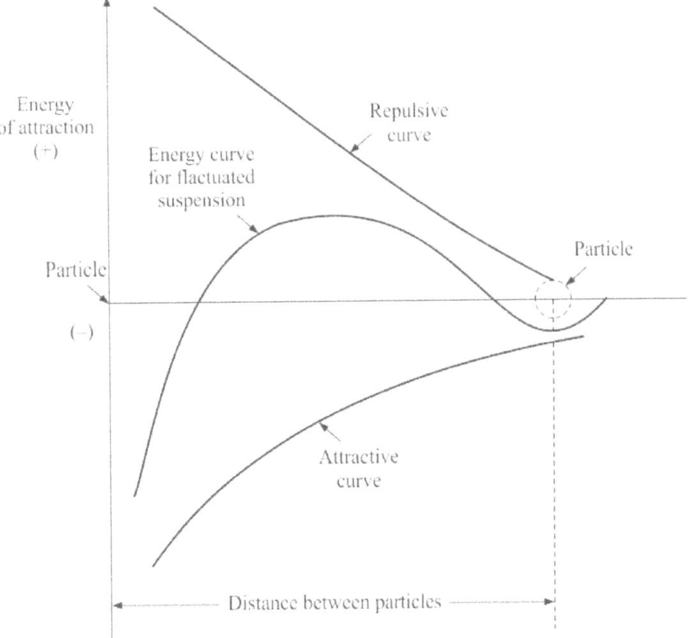

Fig. 8.1(a) Potential energy curves for particle interactions in suspension.

Conclusion:

(a) Flocculated particles are weakly bonded, settle rapidly, do not form cake and are easily resuspended.

(b) Deflocculated particles settle slowly, forms a sediment which results in hard cake.

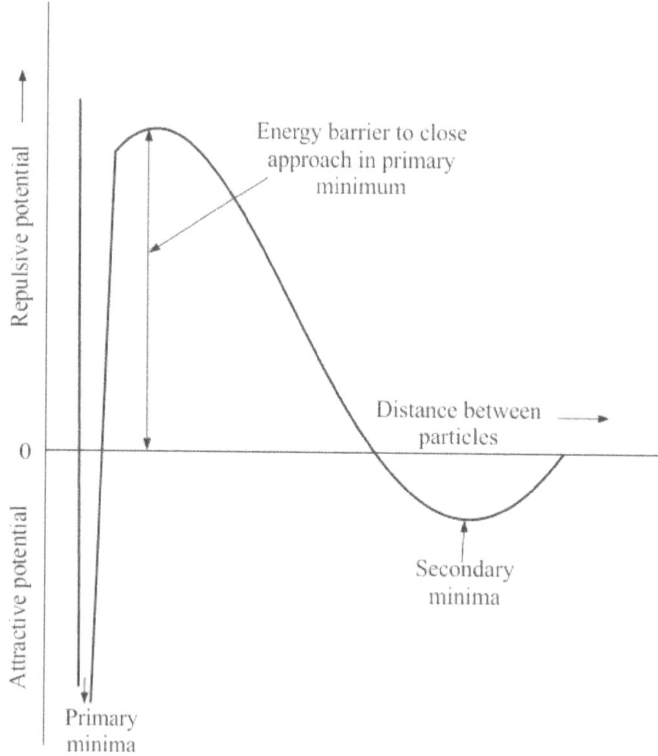

Fig. 8.1(b) Variation in net potential of interaction arising from the combined effects of repulsive and attractive forces between two approaching coarse particles.

8.3   Theory of Sedimentation

The velocity of sedimentation is described by the stoke's law,

$$V = \frac{d^2(\rho_s - \rho_o)g}{18\,\eta_0} \qquad\qquad .....(8.2)$$

where,   V = terminal velocity in cm/sec

d = diameter of the particle in cm

ρ_s = density of dispersed phase

ρ_0 = density of dispersion medium

g = acceleration due to gravity

η_0 = viscosity of the dispersion medium in 'poise'

In dilute suspensions, the particles do not interfere with one another during sedimentation, and free settling occurs. When suspensions have solids in concentration of 5%, 10% or higher concentrations, the particles exhibit hindered setting. The particles interfere with one another as they fall, and stokes law no longer applies.

To account for the non-uniformity in particle shape and size invariably encountered in real systems. We can write stoke's equation in other forms. One of the proposed modification is

$$V^1 = V\varepsilon^n \qquad \qquad .....(8.3)$$

where, V^1 = rate of fall at the interfere in cm/sec

V = velocity of sedimentation according to stokes law

ε = internal porosity

n = exponent is a measure of the 'hindering' of system. It is constant for each system

8.3.1 Effect of Brownian Movement

For particles having a diameter 2 to 5 μm, Brownian movement counteracts sedimentation to a measurable extent at room temperature by keeping the dispersed motion. The critical radius 'r', below which particles will be kept in suspension by kinetic bombardment of the particles by the molecules of the suspending medium (Brownian movement) was worked out by Burton.

It can be seen in the microscope that Brownian movement of the smallest particles in a field of particles of a pharmaceutical suspension is usually eliminated when the sample is dispersed in a 50% glycerine solution, having a viscosity of about 5 centipoise.

8.3.2 Sedimentation Parameters

The two useful parameters that can be derived from sedimentation studies are sedimentation volume, V or height, u and degree of flocculation.

$$\text{Sedimentation volume} \quad F = \frac{V_u}{V_0} \qquad \qquad .....(8.4)$$

V_u = Volume of sediment

V_0 = Original volume of the suspension

F values range from < 1 to > 1. F is normally < 1.

If,

1. The ultimate volume of sediment is smaller than the original volume of suspension then F = 0.5 as per Fig. 8.2 (a).

2. The volume of sediment in a flocculated suspension equals the original volume of suspension then F = 1 as shown in Fig. 8.2 (b).

3. The final volume of sediment is greater than the original when some extra vehicles have been added to contain the sediment then F = 1.5 as per example shown in Fig. 8.2 (c).

If we consider a suspension that is completely "deflocculated" the ultimate volume of the sediment will be relatively small. Writing this volume as V_α based on equation (8.4).

$$F_\alpha = \frac{V_\alpha}{V_0} \qquad \qquad .....(8.5)$$

where,

F_α = the sedimentation volume of the deflocculated, or peptized, suspension.

The degree of flocculation, β is therefore defined as ratio F to F_α or

$$\beta = \frac{F}{F_\alpha} \qquad \qquad .....(8.6)$$

Substituting equations (8.4), (8.5) and (8.6) we obtain

$$\beta = \frac{\frac{V_u}{V_0}}{\frac{V_\alpha}{V_0}}$$

$$\beta = \frac{V_u}{V_\alpha} \qquad \qquad .....(8.7)$$

The degree of flocculation is a more fundamental parameter than F because it relates the volume of flocculated sediment to that in a deflocculated system. We can therefore say that

$$\beta = \frac{\text{Ultimate sediment volume of flocculated suspension}}{\text{Ultimate sediment volume of deflocculated suspension}}$$

8.3.3 Sedimentation behaviour of Flocculated and Deflocculated Suspensions

If the aggregation of the particles in a suspension does occur then the system is said to be flocculated. The nature of flocs will be determined by the closeness of contact of the individual particles.

If the barrier to repulsion is sufficient to prevent aggregation in the primary minimum and the effect of secondary minima is insignificant then the particles will remain as individual units and the system is said to deflocculated.

A flocculated suspension will show a more rapid sedimentation rate than a deflocculated system. The rate of sedimentation in a flocculated system is often referred as subsidence and it depends not only on the size of the aggregates or flocs but also on their porosity, since the liquid medium flows through, as well as around, then as they fall.

In a flocculated suspension loose cake is formed which can redispersed and hard cake is formed in case of deflocculated suspension which do not redisperse easily.

In a deflocculated suspension the repulsive forces between individual particles allow the particles to slip past each other in sediment. This property, together with the slow rate of sedimentation, which prevents the entrapping of liquid medium allows the formation of a compact sediment i.e., one with small volume. This is referred as cake.

In deflocculated suspensions the supernatant solution is cloudy with the presence of small particles but in flocculated suspensions even the small particles are present in the sediment so the supernatant solution is clear.

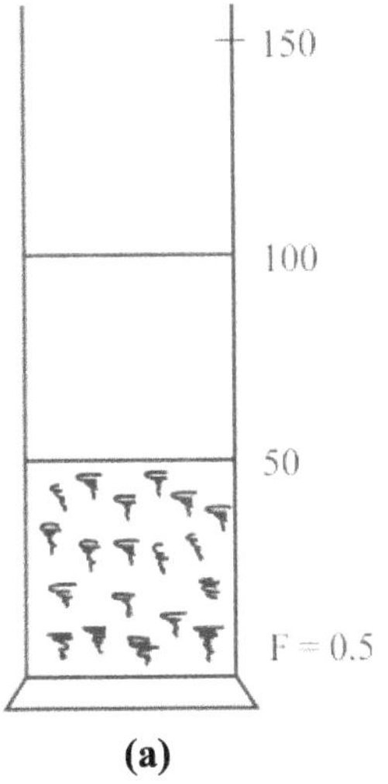

(a)

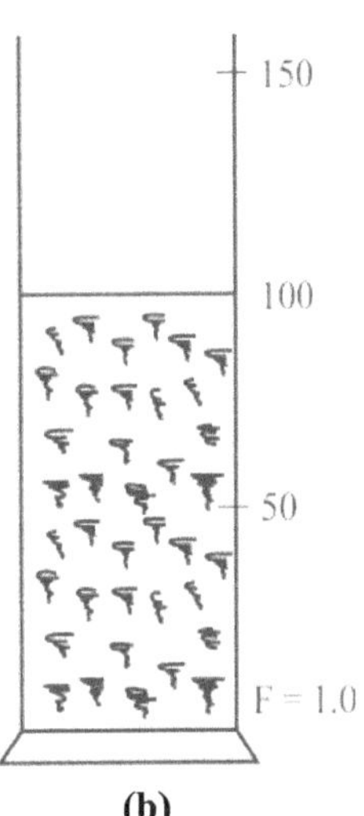

(b)

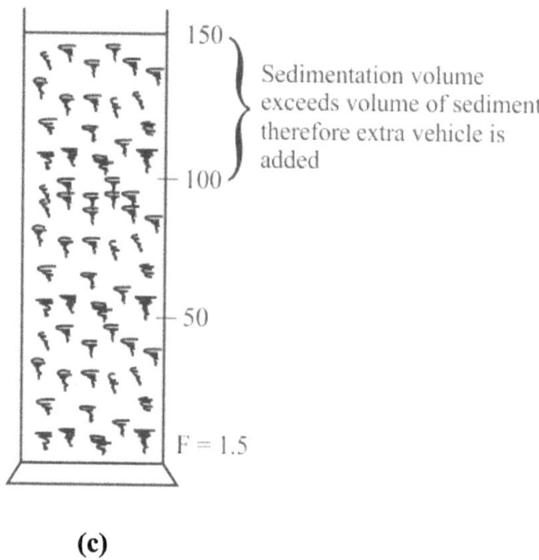

(c)

Fig. 8.2 **(a)** Sedimentation volumes produced by adding varying amounts of flocculating agents, **(b)** and **(c)** are pharmaceutically acceptable.

Period of Floculated Deflocculated Standing

Fig. 8.3 illustrates the difference in appearance of flocculated and deflocculated suspension after various periods of standing in an undisturbed condition.

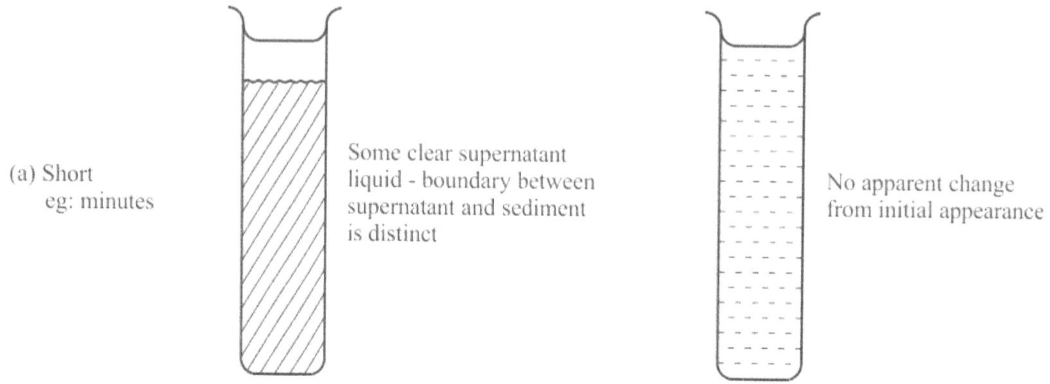

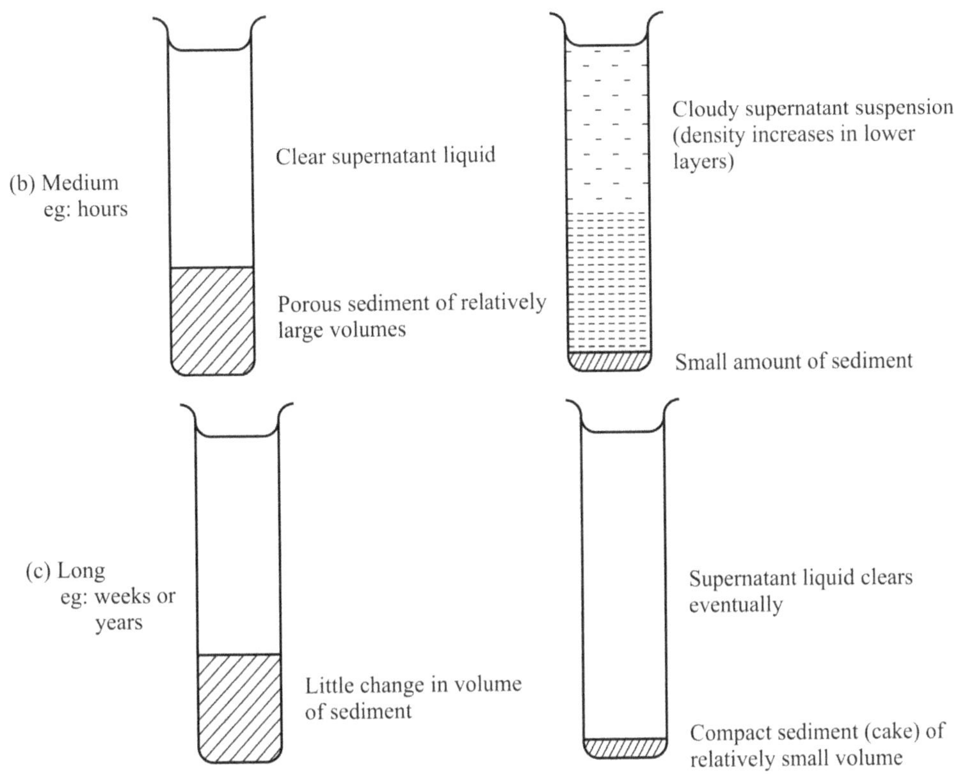

Fig. 8.3 The sedimentation behaviour of flocculated and deflocculated suspensions.

8.4   Formulation of Suspension

During the preparation of physically stable pharmaceutical suspensions, a number of formulation components are used to keep the solid particles in a state of suspension (suspending agents) whereas other components are part of the liquid vehicle itself and have other functions in the dosage form.

8.4.1 Wetting Agents

Wetting agents are surfactants that lower the interfacial tension and contact between solid particles and contact angle between solid particles is added to a liquid vehicle containing a wetting agent, penetration of the liquid phase into the powder will be sufficiently rapid to permit air to escape from the particles. The best range for wetting and spreading by non-ionic surfactants is between a hydrophilic-lipophilic balance (HLB) value of 7 and 10, although surfactants with values higher than 10 are often need for this purpose.

Common wetting agents and surfactants include

   1. Anionic type (docusate sodium and sodium lauryl sulphate).

2. Non-ionic type (polyoxy alkyl ethers, polyonyl alkyl phenyl ethers, polyoxy hydrogenated ester, polyoxy sorbitan esters, and sorbitan esters).

8.4.2 Deflocculants and Dispersing Agents

Unlike surfactants, these agents do not appreciably lower surface and interfacial tension, thus, they have little tendency to create form or wet particles. Most deflocculants, however, are not generally considered safe for internal use, and as a result the only acceptable dispersant for internal products is lecithin or a lecithin derivative (naturally occurring mixture of phosphatides and phospholipids). Because lecithin vary in water solubility and dispersibility characteristics, proper control of product specifications must be maintained to obtain reproducibility.

8.4.3 Flocculating Agents

Primary flocculating agents are simple neutral electrolytes in solution that are capable of reducing the ζ-potential (zeta) of suspended charged particles to zero. Small concentrations (0.01-1%) of neutral electrolytes, such as sodium or potassium chloride, are often sufficient to induce flocculation of weakly charged, water insoluble, organic non-electrolytes. In the case of highly charged, insoluble polymers and polyelectrolyte species, similar concentrations (0.01-1%) of water soluble divalent or trivalent ions, such as calcium salts, alums, sulphates, citrates and phosphates may be required for floc formation, depending on particle charge (positive or negative). These salts are often used together as pH buffers and flocculating agents.

8.4.4 Thickness, Protective Colloids and Suspending Agents

Protective or hydrophilic colloids such as gelatin, natural gums, and cellulosic derivatives, that are adsorbed on insoluble particles, increase the strength of hydration layer formed around suspended particles through hydrogen bonding and molecular interaction. Because these agents do not reduce surface and interfacial tension, they function best in the presence of a wetting agent. Used in low concentration ($< 0.1\%$) as protective colloids and viscosity builders in higher concentration ($> 0.1\%$).

Suspending agents which are commonly used in pharmaceutical suspensions include:

Cellulosic's: Sodium carboxy methyl cellulose, micro crystalline cellulose, methyl cellulose, starch, sodium starch glycolate

Clays:	Attapulgite, bentonite, magnesium aluminium silicate, kaolin, silicon dioxides
Gums:	Acacia, agar, algins, carrageenan, guar, pectin
Polymers:	Carbomers, polyvinyl alcohol, povidone, polyethylene oxide
Sugars:	Dextrin, mannitol, sucrose
Others:	Aluminium monostearate, emulsifying waxes, gelatin

8.5   Emulsions

Particulate systems have been classified on the basis of size into molecular dispersions, colloidal systems and coarse dispersions.

Disperse system may be defined as a system in which one substance (the dispersed phase) is dispersed as particles throughout another (the dispersed medium/continuous phase). They are three types of dispersed systems:

S. No.	Type of system	Dispersed particles	Particle	Notes
1.	True solutions	Small molecules/ions	Usually less than 1×10^{-6} mm	Mixture of gases are restricted to this type of system
2.	Colloidal dispersions	Single large molecules/ions or aggregates of small molecules	Larger than those in true solution and have an upper size limit of about 1×10^{-3} mm	
3.	Coarse dispersions*	Aggregates of molecules	Larger than those in colloidal dispersions	Particle size ranges from about 1×10^{-3} mm to an upper limit which depends on system.

*Suspensions and emulsions come under the coarse dispersions

8.5.1   Definition of Emulsions

An emulsion is a heterogeneous preparation composed of two immiscible liquids (oil and water), one of which is dispersed as fine droplets throughout the other. These are thermodynamically unstable and revert back to separate oil and water phases by fusion/coalescence of droplets unless kinetically stabilised by a third component, the emulsifying agent.

The phase present as small droplets for a period of time is called "Dispersed Phase/Internal phase/ Discontinuous Phase" and the supporting liquid which surrounds it known as "External phase/Continuous phase/Dispersion medium".

The ratio of internal phase volume to the total volume is known as phase volume/phase volume ratio and the internal phase can occupy not more than approximately 74% of total volume of emulsion.

If the internal phase consists of polyhedral rather than spheres then, internal: external phase ratio is altered.

8.6   Types of Emulsions

There are 4 types of emulsions. They are:

1. Oil in Water (O/W) emulsions

2. Water in Oil (W/O) emulsions

3. Multiple emulsions

4. Micro-emulsions

8.6.1 O/W Emulsions

If the oil droplets are dispersed in a continuous aqueous phase, the emulsion is termed as oil-in-water emulsion.

These are administered by all the major parenteral routes. Sterile parenteral oils in water emulsion have been used extensively for the intravenous administration of fats, carbohydrates, vitamins to debilitated patients.

Several oil-in-water emulsion are now available with droplet sizes similar to that of Chylomicrons (0.5-2 μm) the natural fat droplets in the blood that transport ingested fat to lymphatic and circulatory systems.

Medicinal emulsions for oral administration are usually of the oil in water type and require the use of o/w emulsifying agents – such as synthetic non-ionic surfactants, Acacia, Tragacanth and Gelatin.

The bio-availability of oils for absorption may be enhanced when the oil is in the form of small droplets. Furthermore, the absorption of some drugs such as "Griseofulvin" may be enhanced when they are in the form of oil in water emulsion.

Oil in water type of emulsions are less greasy and sticky on application to the skin, will be absorbed more readily because of their lower oil content and can be more easily washed from the skin surface.

Main disadvantage of this type of emulsion is low viscous and tend to cream easily as it consists of low oil concentration.

Oil-in-water emulsions are sometimes made by the phase inversion technique in which the aqueous phase is slowly added to the oil-phase during mixing. Sometimes oil in water type can be changed to water in oil type phase inversion.

8.6.2 W/O Emulsions

If water is the dispersed phase and oil/oleaginous material is the continuous phase, then the system is designated as water in oil types of emulsions.

These are more occlusive and when compared to oil in water type.

It has greasy and exhibits high apparent viscous than oil in water emulsions.

These are used for external application and emulsifiers used are polyvalent soaps, such as calcium palmitate, sorbitan esters, cholesterol and wool fat.

Certain foods such as butter and some salad dressings are water in oil emulsions.

8.6.3 Multiple Emulsions

In these systems both hydrophilic and hydrophobic emulsifiers are used. An oil droplet enclosing a water droplet may be suspended in water to form a water-in-oil in water emulsion (W/O/W). These are formed by non-ionic surfactants.

A water droplet enclosing an oil droplet may be suspended in oil to form a oil in water in oil emulsion (O/W/O). These are called multiple emulsions formed by lipophilic and non-ionic surfactants.

These are of delayed-action drug delivery systems.

These emulsions can also invert however during inversion they usually form simple emulsions.

e.g.: W/O/W emulsion yields an oil in water emulsion.

8.6.4 Micro Emulsions

These are defined as dispersions of insoluble liquids in a second liquid that appear clear and homogenous to the naked eye. These are sometimes called as solubilised systems because on microscopic basis, they seem to behave as true solution. If the small amount of oil is added to an aqueous solution, of a suitable surfactant in the micellar state, the oil may preferentially dissolve in the interior of the micellar because of its hydrophobic character. This is called oil in water micellar solution.

Similarly water in oil solubilisation – especially by a non-ionic surfactant has been attributed to existence of swollen micelles. In these systems, sometimes called reverse micellar solutions, water molecules are found in the polar central portion of a surfactant micelle, the non-polar portion of which is in contact with the continuous lipid phase.

A third type of emulsion (Micro) is formed by ionic surfactants in the presence of co-surfactants (Pentanol dioxyethylene cyclohexane) with hydrocarbons (hexadecane) and water.

8.7   Identification of Emulsions

Several methods are available for testing emulsion type. They are:

1. Dilution method

2. Dye-solubilisation method

3. Conductivity test

4. Fluorescence test

5. $COCl_2$/Filter paper

1. **Dilution Test:** It involves placing a little of the emulsion in water. If the emulsion readily disperses it is o/w, otherwise a w/o type is indicated.

Thick oil in water creams may require slight agitation but usually emulsion type is readily observed as lumps of oil in water cream appear dull in water where as w/o creams are shiny and usually float to the top.

Observation: Emulsion can be diluted only with external phase.

Comments: Useful for liquid emulsions only.

2. **Dye Solubilisation Method:** This method involves during a small amount of water-soluble dye, such as methylene blue on the surface. Rapid dye diffusion indicates that water is the external phase.

   By dusting an oil-soluble dye such as scarlet-red on another part of the emulsion surface dye diffusion for this then indicates contact with oil as in case of w/o emulsions, but for this test to be valid, the top surface of the emulsion be removed otherwise colouration may merely indicate a thin film on top of an oil in water emulsion due to contamination from manufacturing equipment. Alternatively, it indicates an unstable oil in water emulsion.

3. **Conductivity Test:** This method is based on the ability of water to conduct electricity. If the water is the continuous phase, then the emulsion conducts electricity. If oil is the continuous phase, the emulsion fails to fail conduct.

4. **Fluorescence Test:** Since oils fluorescence under UV light, o/w emulsions exhibit dot pattern, w/o emulsion exhibit fluorescence throughout the emulsion.

   It is not always applicable.

5. **$COCl_2$ Filter Paper**

   1. If a drop of emulsion is placed on a filter paper the external phase will tend to spread quickly if it is aqueous. The filter paper wetting method is useless for thick o/w creams or for emulsions of water in thin oils which themselves spread.

   2. Filter paper impregnated with $COCl_2$ and dried (Blue) changes to pink when o/w emulsion is added.

It may fail when emulsion is unstable or breaks in presence of electrolyte.

8.8 Formulation of Emulsions

The formulatory requirements for emulsions are:
   1. Raw Material
   2. Emulsifying Agents
   3. Buffers
   4. Density Modifiers
   5. Humectants

6. Antioxidants

7. Preservatives

8. Flavours, Colours and Sweetening Agents

8.8.1 Raw Materials

The raw materials required for the preparation are collected. These are grouped on the basis of their solubilities in the aqueous and non- aqueous phases. Then, type of emulsion required is determined. Examples – castor oil, liquid paraffin etc.

8.8.2 Emulsifying Agents

The first step in preparation of stable emulsion is selection of the emulsifiers. In order to stabilize the emulsion, these are used. The process of coalescence can be reduced to insignificant level by adding the emulsifying agents.

Ideal Requirements

1. These should be compatible with all formulation ingredients and active pharmaceutical ingredients.

2. These should be stable, non-ionic.

3. It should maintain the stability of the emulsion for the intended shelf life of the product.

   Emulsifiers have a hydrophilic portion and a lipophilic portion with one or the other being more or less pre-dominant.

   Griffith devised a method whereby emulsifying are classified on the basis of hydrophilic-lipophilic balance (HLB) value.

4. It should reduce surface tension to below 10 dynes/cm.

5. It should impart to the droplets an adequate electrical potential so that mutual repulsion occurs

6. It should increase the viscosity of an emulsion.

7. It should be effective in a low concentration.

8. It should be absorbed quickly around the dispersed drops as condensed, non-adherent film that will prevent coalescence.

Choice of an Emulsifying Agent

Toxicity and Irritancy Considerations: The choice of emulgent used will depend not only on its emulsifying ability, but also on its route of administration and on its toxicity. An approved list of emulsifiers as food additives for use in the European Union would be suitable for internally used pharmaceutical emulsions. The regulations mainly include naturally occurring materials and their semi-synthetic derivatives such as polysaccharides as well as glycerol esters, cellulose ethers, sorbitan esters and polysorbates.

Most of these are non-ionic and have a tendency to be less irritant and less toxic than their anionic and cationic.

The concentration of ionic emulsifying agents necessary for emulsification will be irritant to the GI tract and have a laxative effect. So, these are not used for oral emulsions.

For parenteral preparations – non-ionic materials are used such as lecithin, polysorbate 80, methyl cellulose, gelatin and serum albumin.

HLB Method: A useful method has been devised for calculating the relative quantities of emulgents necessary to produce the most physically stable emulsion for a particular oil/water combination. This is called HLB method. It is applied to non-ionic and ionic type of emulgents.

Griffith developed a scale based on the balance of hydrophilic and lipophilic tendencies of surface active emulsifying agents. This is called HLB scale.

If the emulsifiers become more hydrophilic, its solubility in H_2O increases and o/w form is favoured. W/O emulsions are favoured with more lipophilic emulsifiers.

HLB values extend from 1 to 50. HLB value is the indication of substance polarity which vary from 40 for sodium acryl sulphate to 1 oleic acid.

HLB values:

1 to 3	: Antifoaming agents
7 to 10	: Good wetting property
13 to 20	: Solubilisers
13 to 15	: Detergents

Oil in water : HLB value 3 to 16

Water in oil: HLB value 3 to 8

Non-ionic surfactant are effective over pH range of 3 to 10; cationic surfactants are effective over pH range of 3 to 7; anionic surfactants are effective over pH range of greater than 8.

Classification of Emulsifying Agents

The inclusion of an emulsifying agent is necessary to facilitate actual emulsification during manufacture and to ensure emulsion stability during shelf life of product.

HLB values of selected Emulsifiers

Chemical designation	HLB	Water dispensability
Ethylene glycol distearate	1.5	No dispersion
Sorbitan tristearate	2.1	
Propylene glycol monostearate	3.4	
Sorbitan sesquioleate	3.7	
Glyceryl mono-stearate (non-self emulsifying)	3.8	Poor dispersion
Propylene glycol monolaurate	4.5	
Sorbitan monostearate	4.7	
Diethylene glycol monostearate	4.7	
Glyceryl monostearate (Self-emulsifying)	5.5	
Diethylene glycol monolaurate	6.1	Milky dispersion (not stable)
Sorbitan monopalmitate	6.7	
Polyoxyethylene lauryl ether	9.5	Milky dispersion (stable)
Polyoxy ethylene cetyl ether	10.3	
Polyoxyethyle sorbitan stearate	10.5	Translucent to clear dispersion
Polyoxyethylene lauryl phenol	13.0	
Sodium oleate	18.0	Clear solution
Potassium oleate	20.0	
Sodium lauryl sulphate	40	

These forms an adsorbed film around the dispersed droplets between the two phases.

There are many types of emulgent available. But for convenience, these are divided into two main classes.

1. Synthetic and semi-synthetic surface active agents

2. Naturally occurring materials and their derivatives

1. Synthetic and Semi-synthetic Agents: These are divided into four categories.

   1. Anionic

   2. Cationic

   3. Non-ionic

   4. Amphoteric depending on their ionisation in aqueous solutions

2. Naturally occurring materials and their derivatives: These are not used widely. In many instances these surfactants require the presence of an auxiliary non-ionic emulgent in order to form a complex mono-molecular film as o/w interface.

Synthetic and Semi-synthetic Agents

Anionic-Surfactants: In aqueous solutions, these compounds dissociate to form negatively charged anions that are responsible for their emulsifying ability. These are widely used because of their cheapness and because of non toxicity, these are used for external preparations.

E.g.: Alkali metal and Ammonium soaps

Emulgents consist of sodium, potassium or ammonium salt of long-chain fatty acids, such as sodium stearate $C_{17}H_{35}COO^- Na^+$; they produce stable oil and water emulsions, but in some case require an auxiliary non-ionic emulsifying agent.

These will precipitate out as the free fatty acids in acidic solution, so they are more efficient in alkaline medium. These are formed by reacting with an alkali such as potassium, sodium or ammonium hydroxide with fatty acid.

E.g.: Oleic acid + Ammonia – Soap responsible for stabilising white liniment.

These are incompatible with polyvalent cations, which cause phase reversal. So, deionised water is used in their preparation.

Soaps of Divalent and Trivalent materials: Calcium salts are commonly used. These are formed by interacting of the fatty acid with calcium hydroxide.

E.g.: Oleic acid reacted with calcium hydroxide to form calcium oleate used for zinc cream BP and oily calamine lotion. These produce only w/o emulsion.

Amine Soaps: Number of amines will form salts with fatty acids.

E.g: Triethanolamine $N(CH_2CH_2OH)_3$ used in pharmaceutical and cosmetic products.

Triethanolamine stearate forms stable o/w emulsion and usually made *in situ* by reaction between triethanolamine and fatty acid.

Sulfated and Sulfonated Compounds: The alkyl sulphates have general formula $KOSO_3M^-$

R: Hydro carbon chain

M: Sodium or ethanolamine

E.g.: Sodium lauryl sulphate: o/w emulsion. It is used with cetosteryl alcohol to produce emulsifying wax – in order to stabilize aqueous cream and Benzyl Benzoate application. These are less widely used.

Cationic Surfactants: In aqueous solutions these dissociate to form positively charged cations that provide emulsifying preparation.

Important class in Quaternary Ammonium compounds: These are used not for emulsifying preparation but also for preservative preparation.

Disadvantages: Toxicity. So these are used in antiseptic cream only.

E.g.: Cetrimide – 0.5% concentration in cetrimide cream with 5% alcohol.

Non-ionic Surfactants: These products range from oil-soluble compounds stabilizing w/o emulsions to water soluble materials giving oil in water products.

Widely used because of their low toxicity and irritancy. So, used for oral and parenteral administration.

Great degree of compatibility with anionic and cationic emulgents.

To reduce the tendency for coalescence to occur in an o/w emulsion, it is necessary that the polar groups be well dehydrated/sufficiently large to prevent close approach of the dispersed droplets in order to compensate for lack of charge.

Most Non-ionic surfactants are based on:

1. Fatty acid/alcohol (12-18 'c' atoms) – the hydrocarbon chain of which provides the hydrophobic moiety.

2. An alcohol (OH)/ethylene oxide grouping (OCH_2CO_2) – hydrophilic part of molecule.

E.g.: Glycol and glycerol esters.

Glyceryl monosterate produces weak water in oil emulsions. The addition of small amounts of Na^+, K^+ or triethanolamine salts of suitable fatty acids produce self-emulsifying glyceryl monosterate.

Self-emulsifying monostearin is glycerol monosterate to which anionic soaps added. This is used to stabilize hydrocortisone lotion.

Diethylene glycol monostearate, Propylene glycol monoacetate.

Sorbitan Esters: Produced by esterification of one or more hydroxyl groups of sorbitan with either lauric, oleic palmitic or stearic acids. These exhibits lipophilic preparation and form water in oil emulsions. These are used with polysorbates to produce oil in water/water in oil emulsions.

Polysorbates: Polyethylene glycol derivatives of sorbitan esters are polysorbates.

E.g.: Variations in the type of fatty acid used and in the number of oxyethylene groups in polyethylene glycol chains produce a range of products differing in oil in water solubilities.

E.g.: Polyoxyethane 20 sorbitan mono-oleate, polysorbate 80.

Fatty alcohol polyglycol ethers: Condensation products of polyethylene glycol and fatty alcohol (usually cetyl or cetostearly)

$$ROH + (CH_2CH_2O)_n \rightarrow RO(CH_2CH_2O)_n\,H$$

$$R + \text{fatty alcohol chain}$$

E.g.: Macrogol cetostearyl ether or cetomacrogol 1000 – which is polyethylene glycol mono acetyl ether – oil in water emulgent celomarc emulsifying ointment includes celomarcrogol 1000 and cetosteryl alcohol and used to stabilize celomarcrogol cream.

Fatty Acid Polyglycol Esters: Stearate esters or polyoxyl stearates – widely used.

E.g.: Polyoxyethylene 40 stearate oil and water emulsion.

Poloxalcoids: Polyoxyethylene/Polyoxypropylene co-polymers

$$OH(C_2H_4O)_a \ (C_3H_6O)_B \ (C_2H_4O)_a$$

Higher Fatty Alcohols:

E.g.: Hexadecyl and Octadecyl members of this series of saturated mono-hydric alcohols are useful auxiliary emulgents.

Amphoteric Surfactants:

E.g.: Ammonium carboxylates, Ammonium phosphates.

Natural Type of Emulsifying Agents

These are derived from vegetable sources and include acacia, tragacanth, alginates, chondrus, xanthan and pectin. These are forms hydrophilic colloids when added to water and produce oil in water emulsion.

These achieve the emulsifying power by increasing the viscosity of aqueous phase.

From Animal Sources: These are used for both oral and topical preparations

E.g.: Gelatin, Egg yolk, Casein, wool fat, cholesterol, wax and lecithin.

Some of these materials, polysaccharides and protein provide good culture medium for microorganism. So, preservation is necessary. To overcome this, wool fat derivatives and semi-synthetic cellulose such as methyl cellulose and SCMCs are used.

These are mostly used as auxiliary emulsifying agents/stabilizers.

Acacia: Carbohydrate gum soluble in water and forms oil in water emulsions.

Emulsions prepared with acacia are stable over a wide pH range.

Preservative should be added to the emulsion containing acacia as emulgent.

Gelatin: It has two isoelectric points, depending upon the method of preparation.

So called Type A gelatin derived from an acid treated precursor has an iso-electric point between 7 and 9.

Type B gelatin obtained from an alkali-treated precursor having isoelectric point around 5 pH.

Type A gelatin acts as a (emulgent gelatin) around pH 4.7 and Type B gelatin acts as a emulgent around pH 8.

Type A is positively charged at pH 3 and Type B positively charged at pH 8.

Thus if gums such as tragacanth, acacia or agar that are negatively charged are to be used with gelatin, then Type B used as it is positively charged.

Lecithin: It is obtained from plant e.g., soyabean and animal (egg, egg yolk) and is composed of phosphatides.

The important component in this is phosphatidylcholine. But, lecithins contains mixtures of phosphatidylserine, phosphatidylinositol, phosphatidyl ethanolamine and phosphatidic acid in addition to phosphatidylcholine.

It is a zwitterion compound. It is a good emulsifier for naturally occurring oils such as soy, corn or safflower. Highly oil in water emulsions can be formed with these oils. These are principle emulsifiers for intrallenous fat emulsion.

It provides stable emulsion with droplet size of less than 1 μm in diameter. It provides better emulsion at pH 8.

Cholesterol: Major constituent of wool alcohols, obtained by the saponification and fractionation of wool fat. It forms water in oil emulsion.

Finely Dispersed Solids: These form particulate films around the dispersed droplets producing emulsions that are coarse-grained and have considerable physical stability.

Bentonite: White to grey, colourless and tasteless powder and swells in presence of water to form translucent suspensions with pH 9.

Depending upon sequence of mixing, it forms oil in water or water in oil emulsions.

If oil in water emulsion is desired, Bentonite is first dispersed in water and oil phase is added gradually with stirring; for water in oil emulsion, Bentonite is dispersed in oil phase and water is then added gradually.

Veegum: It is used as a stabilizer in cosmetic lotions and creams. Concentration of less than 1% will stabilize an emulsion containing anionic/non-ionic emulsifying agents.

E.g.: Al. Mg. Silicate   – external use

Colloidal $SiO_2(OH)_3$ and $Mg(OH)_2$ – internal use

8.8.3 Buffers

These maintain chemical stability, control toxicity or ensure physiological compatibility. Addtion of electrolyte have prefound effects on stability of emulsions.

8.8.4 Density Modifiers

From qualitative examination of Stoke's law, if the disperse and continuous both have same densities then sedimentation or creaming will not occur. Minor modifications to the aqueous phase of an emulsion occurs by incorporating dextrose, glycerol or propylene glycol can be achieved. Because of different coefficients of expansion, this is possible over a small temperature range.

8.8.4 Humectants

Glycerol, poly ethylene glycol and propylene glycol are examples that are incorporated at a concentration of about 5% into aqueous solution of emulsion for external application.

These are added to reduce the evaporation of water either from the packaged product when the closure is removed from the surface of skin after application. High concentration if used topically, may actually remove moisture from the skin, thereby dehydrating it.

8.8.5 Antioxidants

Before including an antioxidant in emulsion, it is essential to ensure that its use is not restricted in which country it is desired to sell the product. In Briton, BHA (butylated hydroxyl anisole) is widely used for the protection of field oils and fats at concentration of 0.02%and for oils 0.1%.

BHT (Butylated hydroxyl toulene): It is used as an alternative to tocopherol at a concentration of 10 ppm to stabilise liquid paraffin. Other examples – Propyl, octyl and dodecyl esters of gallic acid - 0.001% concentration for fixed oils and fats and 0.1% for essential oils.

Efficiency of Anti-oxidant depends upon

1. Compatibility with other ingredients
2. Oil in water partition coefficient
3. Extent of its solubilisation within micelles of emulsion
4. Its sorption onto the container and closure.

8.8.6 Preservatives

Emulsions are formulated to resist microbial attack, due to this effect physicochemical properties of formulation causing colour, odour and pH changes and phase separation also. Water in oil emulsions are less susceptible to attack than oil in water emulsion because aqueous continuous phase produce ideal condition for growth of bacteria.

Preservatives are not used in parenteral preparation which are sterilized by autoclaving.

The preservative should be free from toxic, irritant and sensitising activity.

Example of preservatives in oral and topical preparations includes:

1. Phenoxyethanol

2. Benzoic acid

3. Parabenzoates

4. Chlorocresol

pH should be considered while adding these preservatives. Problems arise because many of materials used in formulation and hydrocolloids or polyoxyethylene surfactant interact with surfactants thus depleting their activity.

8.8.7 Flavours, Colours and Sweetening Agents

Adsorption of materials onto the surfaces of disperse phase of a suspension may occur, and because of high surface area of dispersed powders in this type of formulation, their effective concentration in solution may be significantly reduced. The final the degree of sub-division of disperse phase, the paler may appear the colour of product for a given concentration of dye. But inclusion of these may alter the physical characteristics of emulsion.

Different high concentrations of sucrose, sorbitol and glycerol are used as sweetening agents. Synthetic sweeteners are also used.

Some of the flavours used are peppermint oil, cinnamon water, etc.

8.9   Physical Insolubility of Emulsions

The stability of a pharmaceutical emulsion is characterised by absence of coalescence of internal phase, absence of creaming, and maintenance of elegance with respect to appearance, odour, colour and other physical properties.

Creaming resulting from flocculation and concentration of globules of internal phase, sometimes is not considered as mark of instability. Creaming results in lack of uniformity of drug distribution and unless it is thoroughly shaken before administration leads to variable dosage.

Phase inversion is one of the problems which involve change of emulsion from oil in water to water in oil or vice versa.

Instability of Emulsions can be classified as:

1. Creaming

2. Flocculation

3. Coalescence

4.   Breaking and

5. Phase inversion

8.9.1 Creaming

Many emulsions forms cream on standing the dispersed phase, according to its density relative to that of continuous phase, rises to the top or sinks to the bottom of emulsion, forming a layer of more concentrated emulsion.

E.g.: Milk – an oil in water emulsion with cream rises to top of emulsion.

The greater the difference between the density of two phases, the larger the oil globules and less viscous the external phase, the greater the rate of creaming.

Droplets of the creamed layer do not coalescence, as may be found by gentle shaking which redistributes the droplet throughout the continuous phase.

The factors that influence the rate of creaming are similar to those involved in sedimentation rate of suspension particles and are indicated by Stoke's law as follows:

$$v = \frac{2a^2 g(\sigma - \pi)}{9\eta}$$

where, v = velocity of creaming

a = globule radius

σ and π = densities of dispersed phase and medium

η = viscosity of dispersion medium

Rate of creaming reduced by:
1. Reduction in the globule size
2. Decrease in density difference between the two phases
3. Increase in viscosity of continuous phase

A rise of creaming rate may therefore be achieved by homogenising the emulsion to reduce the globule size and increasing the viscosity of continuous phase η by the use of thickening agents – tragacanth and methyl cellulose.

8.9.2 Flocculation

Flocculation of the dispersed phase may take place before during or after creaming.

Definition: Reversible aggregation of droplets of internal phase in the form of three dimensional clusters. Flocculation is influenced by the charges on the surface of emulsified globules.

In the absence of protective barrier at interface and if insufficient amount of emulsifier is present, emulsion droplets aggregates and coalesce rapidly.

It occurs only when mechanical/electrical barrier is sufficient to prevent droplet coalescence. It differs from coalescence by the fact that interfacial film and individual droplets remain intact. The reversibility of this type of aggregation depends on strength of interaction between particles, phase volume ratio and concentration of dissolved substances especially electrolytes and ionic emulsifiers.

A high internal phase volume be tight packing of dispersed phase tends to promote flocculation.

Avoidance: It is the secondary minimum occurs readily and can't be avoided. Redispersion can easily be achieved by shaking. Primary minimum flocculation is more serious and re-dispersion is not so easy.

The presence of high density on the dispersed droplets will ensure the presence of high energy barrier and then reduce the flocculation on primary minimum.

Agitation of the emulsion breaks the particle-particle interaction with a resulting drop of viscosity i.e., shear thinning a flocculation, emulsion viscosity are closely related because viscosity of emulsion depends to a large extent on flocculation which restricts the movement of particles.

8.9.3 Coalescence

It is a growth process during which the emulsified particles join to form larger particles. The coalescence of oil globules in an oil in water emulsion is resisted by presence of mechanically adsorbed layer of emulsifier around each globule. This is achieved by presence of either a condensed mixed monolayer of lipophilic and hydrophilic emulgents or multimolecular film of a hydrophilic material.

Hydration of either of these types of films will hinder the drainage of water from between adjacent globules which is necessary prior to coalescence. As two globules approach each other, their close proximity causes their adjacent surfaces to flatten. As a change from a sphere to any other shape results in increase in surface area and hence in total surface free energy; this globule distortion will be resisted and drainage of film of continuous phase between the two globules will be delayed.

The major factor which prevents coalescence in flocculated and unflocculated emulsions is strength of interfacial barrier.

Good shelf life and absence of coalescence can be achieved by formation of a thick interfacial film from manomolecules or from particulate solids. This is the reason a variety of natural gums and proteins are so useful as auxiliary emulsifiers when used at low levels but can even be used as ρ emulsifiers at higher concentration.

Presence of long, corrosive hydrocarbon chains projecting into the oil phase will prevent coalescence in a water in oil emulsion.

8.9.4 Breaking

This is indicated by complete seperation of oil and aqueous phases. It is an irreversible process. In breaking the protective sheath around the globules is completely destroyed.

8.9.5 Phase Inversion

An emulsion is said to be invert when it changes from an oil in water to water in oil emulsion or vice versa.

It is due to:

1. Addition of opposite electrolyte
2. By changing the phase-volume ratio

E.g.: Oil in water emulsion having sodium stearate as the emulsifier can be inverted by the addition of $CaCl_2$ because calcium stearate formed is a lipophilic emulsifier and favours the formation of water in oil product.

Viscosity Changes

Many factors influence the viscosity of emulsions. Any variation in globule size or number or in orientation/migration of emulsifier over a period of time may be detected by changed in apparent viscosity. Suitable method and equipment are used to determine this.

By using the Brookefield viscometer with Helipath stand, can give an indication of change in structure of system after various storage times.

8.10 Stress Conditions for Evaluating Stability of Emulsions

8.10.1 Aging and Temperature

It is used to determine the shelf life of all types of preparations by storing them for various periods of time at temperatures that are higher than those normally encountered. The Arrhenius equation, which predicts that a 10 °C increase in temperature doubles the rate of most chemical reaction, is not applicable to emulsion. Many emulsions may be perfectly stable at 40 or 45 °C, but can't tolerate temperatures in excess of 55 or 60 °C even for a few hours. A particularly useful means of evaluating shelf life is cycling between two temperatures. Again, extremes should be avoided and cycling should be conducted between 4 and 45 °C. Thin type of cycling approaches realistic shelf conditions, but places the emulsion under enough stress to alter various emulsion parameters.

The normal effect of aging an emulsion at elevated temperature to acceleration of rate of creaming/coalescence and this is usually coupled with changes in viscosity.

Most emulsions become thinner at elevated temperatures and thicken when allowed to come to room temperature.

This thickening can be expensive if the emulsion is not agitated during cooling cycle; sometimes the low viscosity can be 'frozen' into the emulsion if it is chilled rapidly.

Freezing can damage an emulsion more than heating, since the solubility of emulsifiers both in lipid and aqueous phase is more sensitive to freezing than to modest warming. Formation of ice crystals develops pressure that can deform the spherical shape of emulsion droplets.

8.10.2 Centrifugation

Shelf life under normal storage conditions can be predicted rapidly by observing the separation of the dispersed phase due to either creaming or coalescence when the emulsion is exposed to centrifugation.

Becher indicates that centrifugation at 3750 rpm in 10 cm – radius centrifuge for a period of 5 hr is equivalent to the effect of gravity for about one year. The modest speed suggested by Becher is reasonably. On other hand the ultra centrifugation at extremely high speeds at 25,000 rpm can cause effects that are not observed during normal aging of an emulsion.

Ultracentrifugation creates 3 layers

1. A top layer of coagulated layer
2. Intermediate layer of uncoagulated emulsion
3. Essentially pure aqueous layer

Rapid formation of clear oily layer is the first clue to 'abnormal' phenomenon taking place during ultracentrifugation.

Force of ultracentrifugation does not cause oil separation until it is high enough to break or rupture the absorbed layer of emulsifier that surrounds each droplet.

8.10.3 Agitation

Droplets in an emulsion exhibit Brownian movement. No coalescence of droplets takes place unless droplets impinge upon each others owing to their Brownian movement.

Simple mechanical agitation can contribute to the energy with which two droplets impinge upon each other. Excessive shaking of an emulsion or excessive homogenisation may interfere with the formation of emulsion.

Agitation can also break emulsions

E.g.: Manufacturing of butter from milk.

Some clear micro emulsions become cloudy upon short agitation in a blender due to coalescence of particles.

Conventional emulsions may deteriorate from gentle rocking on a reciprocating shaker. This is related to in part to impingement of droplets and in part due to reduction of viscosity of normal thixotropic system.

8.10.4   Phase Separation

The rate and extent of phase separation after aging of an emulsion may be observed visually or by measuring the volume of separated phase.

Simple means of determining phase separation due to creaming or coalescence in apparently withdrawing small specimens of emulsion from top and bottom of preparation after some period of storage and comparing the composition of two samples by appropriate analysis of water contents oil contents or any suitable constituent.

8.10.5 Electrophoretic Parameters/Properties

The zeta potential of emulsions can be measured with the aid of moving boundary method or quickly and directly by observing the movement of particles under the influence of electric current.

Zeta potential is essentially for assessing flocculation since electric charges on particles influence rate of flocculation.

Measurement of electrical conductivity is a powerful tool for the evaluation of emulsion stability. It is determined with the aid of electrodes of point for oil in water and water in oil microamperometrically to produce a current of about 15 to 80 μA.

Measurements made on emulsions stored for short periods of time at room temperature 37 °C. Then oil in water preparation with fine particles exhibit low resistance, it is a sign of oil droplet aggregation and instability.

A fine emulsion of water in water in oil product does not conduct current until droplet coagulation i.e., instability occurs.

It can be seen when an emulsion, prepared by heating and mixing the two phases, is being labelled. This takes place presumably because of temperature independent changes in solubilities of emulsifying agents.

The phase inversion temperature (PIT) of non-ionic surfactants has been shown by Shinado and Kunieda to be influenced by the HLB number of surfactant – the higher the PIT value, the greater the resistance to inversion. It is avoided by using the proper emulsifying agent in adequate concentration.

The volume of dispersed phase should not exceed 80% of total volume of emulsion.

8.11   Evaluation and Testing for Emulsions

8.11.1 Methods of Assessing Stability

The final acceptance of emulsion depends on stability, appearance and functionality of the packaged product. The most obvious problems facing the formulator are:

1. What is acceptable shelf life
2. What are the predictive indicators of shelf life

The container used for packaging an emulsion may be expected to a source of incompatibility. So, final evaluation of the product must be conducted in a container that will be used commercially.

To speed up the stability program, the formulator commonly uses the emulsion under some sort of stress condition. Stress condition normally evaluated for stability of emulsions, include aging and temperature centrifugation and agitation.

***Methods used are*:**

1. Microscopic examination
2. Globule size analysis
3. Accelerated stability studies

1. Macroscopic Examination

The   Physical stability can be assessed by an examination of degree of creaming or coalescence occurring over a period of time.

This is carried out by calculating the ratio of volume of creamed or separated part of emulsion and the total volume. These values compared for different products.

2. Globule Size Analysis

If mean globule size increases with time, it can be assumed that coalescence is the cause. It is therefore possible to compare the rates of coalescence for a variety of emulsion formulations by measuring changes in globule size and number.

Microscopic examinations, electronic particle counting devices such as coulter counter and laser diffraction sizing are most widely used.

3. Accelerated Stability Studies

Normally flocculation and creaming are slow processes. however this can be evaluated by centrifugation method. The emulsions are subjected to centrifugal speeds (2000-3000 rpm) at room temperature and the separation of phases is observed at different time periods. A good emulsion does not exhibit detectable separation of oil phase.

8.12   Theories of Emulsification

When oil and water are mixed and agitated, droplets of varying sizes are produced. A tension exists at interface because two immiscible phases tends to have different attractive forces for a molecule at interface.

Greater the degree of immiscibility, greater the interfacial tension.

For liquid hydrocarbons such as mineral oil, exhibit an interfacial tension of 50 dynes/cm against water. For polar vegetable oil, such as olive oil exhibit a value of 23 dynes/cm.

Definition of Interfacial Tension

Interfacial tension at a liquid interface is defined as the work required to create 1 cm^2 of new interface.

A high interfacial free energy favours a reduction of interfacial area, first by causing droplets to assume a spherical shape (minimum surface area) and then by causing them to coalesce.

8.12.1   Droplet Stabilisation

Two conceptual alternatives exist for causing opaque i.e., milky appearing emulsions.

Such dispersions can be formed and stabilised by lowering the interfacial tension or by preventing the coalescing of droplets.

According to classic emulsion theory, surface active agents are capable of performing both objectives. They reduce interfacial tension and they act a barriers to droplet coalesce since they are adsorbed at the interface or on the surface of suspended droplets.

Emulsifying agents assist in formation of emulsions by three mechanisms

1.   Reduction of interfacial tension – thermodynamic stabilisation.
2.   Formation of rigid interfacial film – mechanical barrier to coalescence.
3.   Formation of electrical double layer – electrical barrier to approach of particles.

1.   Reduction of Interfacial Tension

Lowering of interfacial tension is one way in which the increased surface free energy associated with the formation of droplets and hence surface area in an emulsion can be reduced. If the droplets are spherical, then

$$\Delta F = \frac{6\chi v}{d}$$

χ = volume of dispersed phase in millilitres

d = mean diameter of particles

Many polymers and finely divided solids not efficient in reducing interfacial tension, form excellent interfacial barriers act to prevent coalescence and are useful as emulsifying agents.

2. Formation of Rigid Interfacial Film

The major requirement of potential emulsifying agent is that it readily forms around each droplet of dispersed material.

The main purpose of this film - which can be a monolayer, multilayer or a collection of small particles adsorbed at the interface is to form a barrier that prevents coalescence of droplets that come in contact with one another.

For the film to be efficient barrier, it should possess some degree of surface elasticity and should not thin out and rupture when sandwiched between two droplets. If broken, the film should have the capacity to reform rapidly.

Mechanism of Action: Emulsifying agents may be classified in accordance with the type of film at the interface between two phases.

Monomolecular Films: Those surface-active agents that are capable of stabilising an emulsion do so by forming a monolayer of adsorbed molecules or ions at the oil-water interface. In accordance with Gibb's law, the presence of an interfacial excess necessitates a reduction in interfacial tension. This results in more stable emulsion because of a proportional reduction in surface free energy.

If the emulsifier forming the mono-layer is ionised, the presence of strongly charged and mutually repelling droplets increases the stability of system with un-ionised, non-ionic surface active agents, the particles may still carry a charge, this arises from adsorption of a specific ion/ion from solution. Wedge theory proposes that surfactants form mono molecules layer around droplets phase of emulsion.

Multimolecular Films: Hydrated lyophilic colloids forms multi molecular films around droplets of dispersed oil.

Although these hydrophilic colloids are adsorbed at an interface, they do not cause an appreciably lowering in surface tension. Rather, their efficiency depends on their ability to form strong coherent multimolecular films. These act as coating around the droplets and render them highly resistant to coalescence even in the absence of well developed surface potential.

Any hydro colloid not adsorbed at the interface increases the viscosity of continuous aqueous phase this increases emulsion stability.

Solid Particle Films: Small solid particles that are wetted to some degree by both aqueous and non-aqueous liquid phases act as emulsifying agents.

If particles are too hydrophilic, they remain in aqueous phase. If too hydrophobic, they remain in oil phase. A second requirement in that the particles are small in relation to the droplets of dispersed phase.

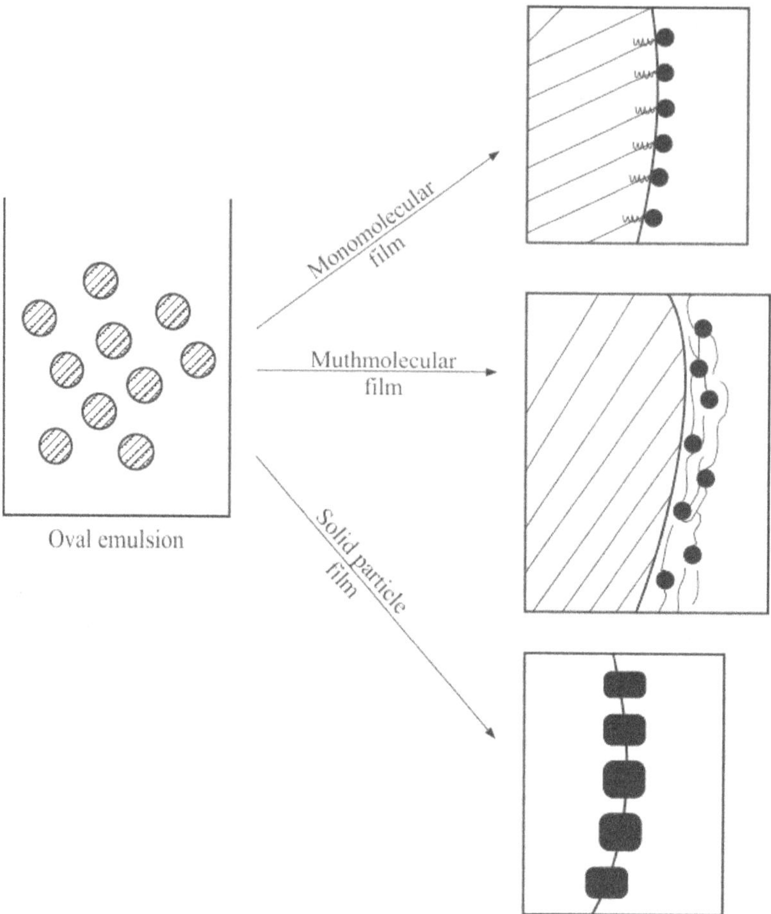

Fig. 8.4 Types of films.

3. Formation of Electrical Double Layer

It describes how interfacial films or lamellar liquid crystals insignificantly alter the rates of coalescence of droplets by acting as barriers. In addition the same similar film can produce repulsive electrical forces between droplets. Such repulsion is due to electrical double layer which may raise from electrically charged groups oriented on the surface of emulsified globules.

The potential developed by the double layer creates a repulsive effect between the oil droplets and thus hinders coalescence. Although, the repulsive electric potential at the emulsion interface can be calculated, it can't be measured directly for comparison with theory. So, zeta potential is determined. The zeta potential for a surfactant stabilised emulsion compares favourably with the calculated double layer potential. In addition the change in double zeta potential parallel rather satisfactorily the change in double-layer potential as electrolyte is added. These and related data on the magnitude of potential at the interface is used to calculate total repulsion between oil droplets as a function of distance between them.

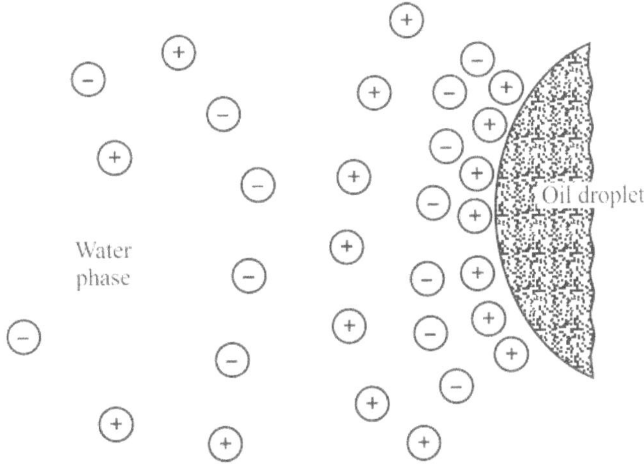

Fig. 8.5 Identical representation of the electrical double layer at an oil in water interface.

8.13 Chemical Instability of Emulsions

It is necessary to ensure that any emulgent system used is not only physically but also chemically compatible with the active agent and with the other emulsion ingredients.

It has been demonstrated that the presence of electrolyte can influence the stability of an emulsion by either.

1. Reducing the energy of interaction between adjacent globules.
2. A salting-out effect, by which high concentrations of electrolytes can strip emulsifying agents of their hydrated layers and so cause their precipitation.

In some cases phase inversion may occur rather than deemulsification.

For Example: A sodium soap is used to stabilize an o/w emulsion, then the addition of a divalent electrolyte such as calcium chloride may form the calcium soap, which will stabilize a w/o emulsion.

Changes in pH may also leads to the breaking of emulsions. Sodium soaps may react with acids to produce the free fatty acid and the sodium salt of the acid. Soap-stabilized emulsions are usually formulated at alkaline pH.

They are three types

1. Oxidation
2. Microbiological contamination
3. Adverse storage conditions

1. *Oxidation*: Many of the oils and fats used in emulsion formulation are of animal or vegetable origin and can be susceptible to oxidation by atmospheric oxygen or by the action of microorganisms. The resulting rancidity is manifested by the formation of degradation products of unpleasant odour and taste. These problems can also occur with certain emulsifying agents, such as wool fat or wool alcohol. Oxidation of microbiological origin is controlled by the use of antimicrobial preservatives, and atmospheric oxidation by the use of reducing agents or antioxidants.

2. *Microbiological Contamination*: The contamination of emulsions by microorganisms can adversely affect the physicochemical properties of the product, causing such as problems as gas production, colour and odour changes, hydrolysis of fats and oils, pH changes in the aqueous phase, and breaking of the emulsion. Even without visible signs of contamination an emulsion can contain many bacteria and, if these include pathogens, may constitute a serious health hazards. Some of the hydrophilic colloids, which are widely used as emulsifying agents, may provide a suitable nutritive medium for bacteria and moulds.

   Species of the genus *pseudomonas* can utilize polysorbates, aliphatic hydrocarbons and compounds. Some fixed oils including arachis oil can be used by some species like *Aspergillus* and *Rizopus*, and liquid paraffin by *penicillium species*.

3. **Adverse Storage Conditions:** Adverse storage conditions may also cause emulsion instability. It has been already explained that an increase in temperature will cause an increase in the rate of creaming, owing to a fall in apparent viscosity of the continuous phase. The temperature increase will also cause an increased kinetic motion, both of the dispersed droplets and of the emulsifying agent at the oil/water interface.

At the other extreme, freezing of the aqueous phase will produce ice crystals that may exert unusual pressures on the dispersed globules and their adsorbed layer of emulgent. In addition, dissolved electrolyte may concentrate in the unfrozen water, thus affecting the charge density on the globules. Certain emulgents may also precipitate at low temperatures. The growth of microorganisms within the emulsion can cause deterioration, so therefore to protect from microorganisms during manufacture, storage and use, and that they contain adequate preservatives.

8.14   Release of Drugs from Emulsion Formulations

The main commercial use of emulsions is for the oral, rectal, and topical administration of oils and oil-soluble drugs. Lipid emulsions are also widely used for intravenous feeding, although the choice of emulgent is very limited and globule size must be kept below four micrometre diameter to avoid the formation of emboli. The high surface area of dispersed oil globules will enhance the rate of absorption of lipophilic drugs. The emulsions can also be used as sustained-release dosage form. The intramuscular injection of certain water-insoluble vaccines formulated as w/o emulsions can provide a slow release of the antigen and result in a greater antibody response and hence a longer lasting immunity on other drugs have also been shown this effect, the rate of release being dependent mainly upon the oil/water partition coefficient of the drug and its rate of diffusion across the oil phase.

It is also possible to formulate multiple emulsion systems in which an aqueous phase is dispersed in oil droplets, which in turn are dispersed throughout another aqueous external phase, producing a water-in-oil-in-water (w/o/w) emulsion. These products can also be used for the prolonged release of drugs that are incorporated in to the internal aqueous phase. They have the advantage of exhibiting a lower viscosity than their w/o counterparts and hence are easier to inject.

Similarly, o/w/o emulsions can be formulated and are also under investigation as potential sustained-release bases. Multiple emulsions, however, tend to be stable only for a relatively short time, although the use of polymers as alternatives to the traditional emulsifying agents may improve their physical stability.